THE DHA STORY

THE DHA STORY

How Nature's Super Nutrient Can Save Your Life

Robert Abel, Jr., M.D.

Basic Health Publications, Inc.

The information contained in this book is based upon the research and personal and professional experiences of the author. It is not intended as a substitute for consulting with your physician or other healthcare provider. Any attempt to diagnose and treat an illness should be done under the direction of a healthcare professional.

The publisher does not advocate the use of any particular healthcare protocol but believes the information in this book should be available to the public. The publisher and author are not responsible for any adverse effects or consequences resulting from the use of the suggestions, preparations, or procedures discussed in this book. Should the reader have any questions concerning the appropriateness of any procedures or preparation mentioned, the author and the publisher strongly suggest consulting a professional healthcare advisor.

Basic Health Publications, Inc.
8200 Boulevard East
North Bergen, NJ 07047
1-201-868-8336

Library of Congress Cataloging-in-Publication Data
Abel, Robert, Jr.
The DHA story : how nature's super nutrient can save your life / Robert Abel, Jr.
p. ; cm.
Includes bibliographical references and index.
ISBN 1-59120-001-6
1. Docosahexaenoic acid—Health aspects. I. Title.
[DNLM: 1. Docosahexaenoic Acids—metabolism—Popular Works. 2. Docosahexaenoic Acids—therapeutic use—Popular Works. 3. Dietary Supplements—Popular Works. WB 425 A141d 2002]
QP752.D63A24 2002
613.2'84-dc21

2002013997

Editor: Stephany Evans
Typesetter/Book design: Gary A. Rosenberg
Cover design: Mike Stromberg

Printed in the United States of America

10 9 8 7 6 5 4 3 2

Contents

Acknowledgments, ix

Foreword, xi

Introduction: DHA—An Essential Building Block of Life, 1

1. The Cell Membrane: Nature's Protective Barrier, 7
2. Cell Biochemistry (or Why the Cat Needs the Mouse), 19
3. DHA: The Cornerstone of Health, 33
4. Healthy Mothers, Healthier Babies: DHA and Pregnancy, 43
5. Sight for Sore Eyes, 51
6. The Brain and Neurologic Health, 71
7. A Matter of Heart, 85
8. Aging Gracefully, 95
9. Building a Better Temple: DHA and Wellness for Life, 105

Glossary, 113

Appendix A: Dietary Sources of DHA, 119

Appendix B: DHA and EPA Supplement Sources, 125

Appendix C: Recommended Reading, 127

References, 129

Index, 139

To my wife, Mike,
and my children,
Ari, Lauren, and Adam.

Acknowledgments

Ted Caddell and Carolyn Zsoldos, R.N., have my deepest appreciation for their collaboration on this project. Their typing and revision skills made this book a reality. Maria Vlasak's careful and kind assistance with structure and syntax made this book readable. And the support I received from Nancy Abel-Hoffenberg; Hack Hoffenberg; Don Willard; Sara Machowski; Ethan Leonard of Martek; Susan Carlson, R.P.H., of Carlson Laboratories; my parents, Robert and Nancy Abel; my aunt Valla Amsterdam; Cheryl Hirsch; and Stephany Evans made this book a joy to write.

I'd like to thank Norman Goldfind, my publisher, for recognizing the importance of DHA for people of all ages and making this book possible. I'd also like to acknowledge David Kyle, Ph.D., whose writings in the field of essential fatty acids sparked my initial interest in DHA, and whose expertise was of invaluable assistance, and the late Steven J. Gould, Ph.D., who pushed back the frontiers in so many scientific fields. Dr Gould's work has had a profound effect on me; his insights and intellect have lit the way for so many of us.

Foreword

As a society, we are starving our children. Yet this newest generation to the planet is so obese that children are developing Type II diabetes in unprecedented numbers at younger and younger ages. In a recent article in the *Wall Street Journal,* the World Health Organization announced that obesity has become a worldwide epidemic even in the world's poorest nations.

How can this be? How can I state that our children are starving and in the very next sentence proclaim that obesity is one of our top health hazards? The answer lies in what we are feeding our children—and also in what we are failing to feed our children. The fast, tasty, easy processed foods that bedeck our glittering food emporia are mostly empty calories that fatten our children while robbing their brains, nervous systems, eyes, and very spirits of the nourishment they need to flourish. And yet, in our fat-phobic obsession to be thin and have slender children, we have labeled all fats as the enemy.

But we need to be far more selective before we seek to banish one-third of all naturally occurring nourishment. Some fats are so important, they are said to be "essential"—essential fatty acids. One of these essential fatty acids is DHA, or docosahexaenoic acid, a nutrient that's critical to the healthy development of the infant brain. DHA is so important to infants' growth and development, in fact, that European nations have been including it in baby formula for years.

Human breast milk is rich in essential fatty acids particularly DHA. When a mother cannot nurse, her baby loses out. In 1994, the World Health Organization began recommending that DHA and another fatty acid called arachidonic acid (ARA) be added to infant formula. The U.S. debut of these products came only after years of scientific debate over the value of supplementing formula with DHA and ARA—two building blocks of the brain and the retina. Proponents point to studies in which supplemented formula, compared with conventional formula, appeared to enhance brain and vision development. Recently, even the FDA (with great reservation) stated that it would allow manufacturers of baby formula to supplement their products with DHA.

"My reading of the literature is there is a clear benefit in neurodevelopment," says Norman Salem of the National Institute on Alcohol Abuse and Alcoholism, who conducted some of the research about the benefits of DHA-supplemented formulas. "My personal opinion is that it [supplementation] should be mandatory."

In this groundbreaking, reader-friendly book, Dr. Robert Abel, Jr., world renowned ophthalmologist, takes us from attention deficit hyperactivity disorder (ADHD) to macular degeneration and deftly makes the case for an "oil change" to DHA-rich foods and supplements. The horizon for DHA supplementation extends literally from conception to advanced old age. Few nutrients perform as many critical functions in all age groups.

I am proud to have been included in Dr. Abel's pioneering efforts to bring research expertise to the public, ensuring the health and well-being of countless individuals and their families. He joins hundreds of integrative practitioners who use nutrition, wise supplementation, and a humane ear to coach patients to wellness and healthy living.

Ronald L. Hoffman, M.D., C.N.S.
President, American College for Advancement In Medicine (ACAM)
Host, Health Talk on WOR Radio
www.drhoffman.com • www.acam.org

INTRODUCTION

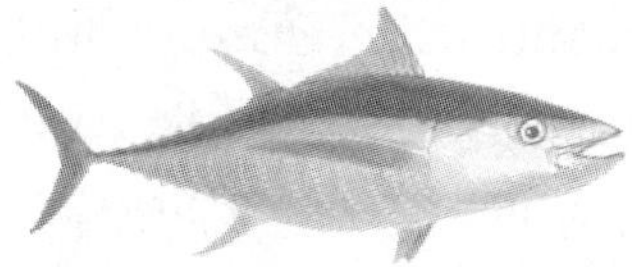

DHA—An Essential Building Block of Life

The great apes of Africa weigh approximately 800 pounds at maturity and have a brain that averages 400 cubic centimeters in volume. In contrast, the human brain is enormous. A 180-pound man has a brain volume of 1,300 to 1,500 cubic centimeters. The reason for this vast difference between our human brains and those of our animal cousins is a little known essential oil called *docosahexaenoic acid*—DHA for short. DHA does not just give our brain "heft." As an omega-3 polyunsaturated fatty acid, it is an important building block of almost every cell in the body.

It is important to get an adequate supply of dietary DHA early in life so that our bodies can grow and develop using the best materials possible. Later in life, DHA is important to maintain strong and healthy cell membranes that maintain their flexibility and can yield without breaking.

WHERE DOES DHA COME FROM?

DHA is abundant in seafood and sea plants, but it is not found in terrestrial plants. We take in DHA first from the milk of our mothers, and later from some of the foods that we eat. Certain animals, such as cows and mice, can convert precursors of DHA found in grass and seeds into DHA itself. But humans cannot do this as efficiently, and must therefore include DHA in our diet from some more immediately accessible form. As I will describe throughout this book, a diet rich in seafood and sea plants is key to having enough of this important essential oil to keep the body and brain running optimally.

DHA AND OVERALL HEALTH

As an ophthalmologist and eye surgeon, I came to realize that often surgery removed only the symptoms that a given patient was experiencing, not the cause. For instance, macular degeneration is a disease that usually strikes older people and leads to a progressive blindness. While some people with the "wet" form of macular degeneration benefit from laser intervention, the disease is usually said to be untreatable. I have spent years studying dietary management for macular degeneration, and I have found that the right nutrients can not only arrest the condition, but can also actually improve it. It turns out that DHA can make a big difference in the eye health of my patients with this degenerative condition. (You'll learn more about the use of DHA to support eye health in detail in Chapter 5.)

I learned that 30 to 50 percent of the building blocks of the membranes of the rods in the retina are DHA, ten times more than any other component in these membranes! The cones, which are in the macula, cannot be studied sufficiently, but scientists assume the same composition ratio exists both in the rods and cones, extremely sensitive cell membranes. DHA, as we'll discuss, is necessary for nerve conduction, so an adequate amount of DHA in the diet is necessary to maintain optimal visual function.

When writing prescriptions for my patients, I began incorporating DHA in a regimen of nutrients—vitamins A and E, lutein, and ginkgo biloba—for improving ocular function. After they began taking the DHA, my patients often reported that their mental status also seemed improved, as well as many of their other vital functions. On my recommendation, a colleague prescribed DHA to a patient of his who had very dry eyes. One month later, the patient returned and congratulated him for being such a fine doctor, because along with improvement to her eyes, she was experiencing less aching in her joints, her bowel function was better, and it seemed to her that even her breast cysts were less painful.

THE IMPORTANCE OF THE ONE-TO-ONE RATIO

Examining DHA and its uses in more detail, I realized that my patients with heart disease and degenerative neurologic disease, as well as depression, often responded dramatically to supplementation. I believe the reason for this is clear. Nutritional experts recommend having a one-to-one ratio of omega-6 and omega-3 fatty acids to maintain optimal mental and physical function, because that is the exact ratio of those essential fatty acids in our brains. This ratio is closer to that of the diet of our early hunter-gatherer ancestors and a long way from the typical ratio of twenty-to-one in our modern diet. Although we get ample amounts of omega-6 fats in our Western diet, we get very little of the omega-3 fats *and almost no DHA.*

Incorporating cold-water fatty fish—such as cod, salmon, mackerel, sardines, or hake—in our diet allows us to regain the one-to-one ratio that is so important for a healthy body and mind. Although seafood is an excellent source of DHA, fish themselves are in the same boat as humans. Neither humans nor fish can make DHA very well, and so we must rely on our diets to provide this essential nutrient. Fish depend upon the tiny phytoplankton (microalgae or microplants) in the sea as a source of DHA. In fact, phytoplankton are ultimately the primary producers of DHA on our planet.

IN THE BEGINNING . . .

As I began to fully appreciate the significance of DHA to our health, I felt drawn to understand how we came to be so dependent on this fatty acid. Interestingly, what I discovered is that DHA is connected to the origin of life itself.

Algae were the first cells on this planet, the sole occupants of the world for approximately 1.6 billion years. These first life forms were able to emerge from the primordial ooze only after they formed protective cell membranes. Because scientists have identified DHA in the eyespots of the most ancient algae found today, it is believed DHA may have been part of those original cell membranes. Eventually, the algae developed *chloroplasts,* intracellular organelles that store chlorophyll, and made enough oxygen through photosynthesis that a new group of organisms evolved: the consumers, or "algae eaters." Oxygen, along with sugars and amino acids were the fuels of life for the consumers. Multicellular life forms, fungi, invertebrates, and animals then eventually evolved and exploded onto the planet. Man, the ultimate consumer, is at the top of the food chain. He eats everything!

You might be wondering why the human body can't efficiently manufacture DHA if it's so important to our health and well-being. One theory is that because *Homo sapiens* evolved as an omnivorous "hunter-gatherer" species, DHA was always in our diet and there was no need to expend the metabolic energy to make it. Because dietary DHA was readily available, natural selection would have favored the gene pool that did not expend energy making something that was normally obtained with no effort. The most successful early *Homo sapiens* could rely on other species to make the DHA for them.

Like everything else, our diet has evolved and changed over time. In the past, these changes often were a consequence of exploration, finding new foods in the New World, and later the industrialization of agricultural food products. However, the most dramatic change in our diet was the result of a seemingly benign invention courtesy of Mr. George Wesson.

Wesson developed the technology that has led to the production of low-cost vegetable oils. As a result of Wesson's processing methods and industrialized high-intensity agriculture, low-cost vegetable oils were made available to the world, and fat consumption skyrocketed. But vegetable oil contains little of the omega-3 fat, and no DHA at all. Thus, DHA quickly evaporated out of our Western diet, and today Americans have the lowest per capita consumption of DHA of any nation in the world.

I am concerned that our traditional Western diet contains too much of the five "white thieves": refined sugar, refined flour, lard, salt, and white rice without bran. These provide only empty calories; calories that lack any nutritional powerhouses such as antioxidants and the essential fats. It may be that the lack of these essential fats, especially DHA, is responsible for the growing incidence of cardiovascular, neurological, and visual disorders in our modern society. Arthritis, dry skin, cardiac arrhythmia, hypertension, depression, osteoporosis, learning disabilities, attention deficit disorder, digestive disabilities, and hyper-aggression all are conditions that are adversely affected by low levels of essential fatty acids such as DHA.

DHA has recently been found to deactivate the enzymes that destroy cartilage. It is effective in decreasing inflammation in general. It supports nerve function, sensory organs, and the ability to learn. It decreases cardiac arrhythmia and muscle spasms, improves bone density, decreases blood triglycerides, improves the ratio of "good" cholesterol to "bad" cholesterol, increases memory, and decreases depression. DHA may perhaps even be used to successfully prevent Alzheimer's disease.

In 1937, the 75th United States Congress recommended nutritional support because of the loss of certain essential nutrients in the soil of America's farmlands. In other words, by the early decades of the last century, it was already known that to maintain optimal health, we must either eat well or supplement our diets with nutrient pills!

Many of us practice at least a smidgen of denial in regard to our state of health. If we are not experiencing a health crisis this very moment, we may consider ourselves to be in "good" health—even if we know that on a daily basis we are not making healthy choices that will support long-term good health. Are we really eating well enough? Are we actively protecting the health of our bodies and our brains? We should all ask ourselves these questions. If we can be proactive in taking care of ourselves, we won't later have to rely on physicians and medications to deal with disease after our bodies begin to break down and symptoms become apparent.

DHA, the amazing nutrient that is the subject of this book, can be a crucial component of your regular self-care. It is one that I guarantee can enhance anyone's well-being and quality of life.

CHAPTER ONE

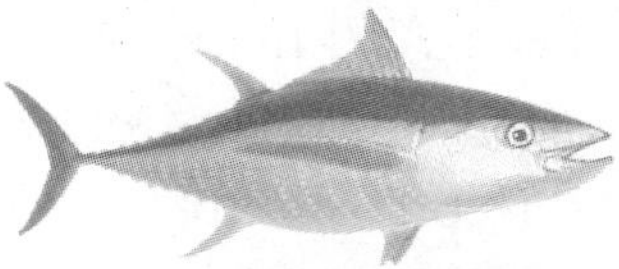

The Cell Membrane: Nature's Protective Barrier

It is the cell membrane that separates organized, internal cellular life from external chaos.

—DOC ABEL

This book is about coming to understand and implement some health basics. In these pages, our discussions will touch upon many nutrients that support human health, but we will always come back to the one that is essential for the health of every one of our cells: *docosahexaenoic acid,* or *DHA.*

We tend to think of genetics as perhaps the newest, most cutting-edge field of study—after all, it was only in 1856 that Gregor Mendel began studies on pea plants that provided the foundation for genetic study, well after the foundations had been laid for other areas of scientific study. But nutrient knowledge is a younger science still. Vitamins, for example, have been recognized only since 1903, when their chemical structure was first determined. Since that time, thousands of studies have confirmed the value of these essential nutrients in the prevention and treatment of many common diseases. Still, it is clearly too early in the game to think that we know all there is to know about nutrients.

In fact, some would say that it's just beginning to get interesting.

We've all heard that "an apple a day keeps the doctor away" and "you are what you eat." And many of us can remember our grandmothers forcing upon us a spoonful of cod liver oil once a day "because it's good for you." You may have thought that these were simply clichés or old wives' tales, but this handful of nutritional aphorisms contain more truth than you might, at first, imagine. Let's start with a look at some basic nutritional building blocks: carbohydrates, fats, and proteins.

THE CHEMICALS OF LIFE

All living things are made up of chemical elements—substances that cannot be broken down into other substances. Our own bodies are composed of carbon, hydrogen, oxygen, nitrogen, sulfur, calcium, phosphorous, and small amounts of other chemicals. To understand how these essential elements affect our body and our health, let's first look at how they were formed.

In the early days of the earth, there were no trees, grasses, or flowering plants. Life evolved only as very small particles called atoms began grouping together. The chemical elements listed above—as well many others that are not mentioned here—are each made up of one kind of atom. Two or more atoms join together to form a molecule; two or more atoms of different elements combine to form complex compounds. Of the compounds found on earth, those containing the element carbon are the most diverse. Many of the everyday things around you are made of carbon chains. If you are not a chemistry major, it's a surprisingly diverse list: the gas you put in your car, the flowers in the garden, and even the plastics that make our everyday lives easier all are made of different kinds of carbon chains. Oh, and besides gas, flowers, and plastic, *butter* would go on that list, too.

Of course, as life evolved on earth, living organisms needed nutrients to sustain themselves. Three major nutritional building blocks are carbohydrates, proteins, and fats. Let's run through a few quick definitions:

- A *carbohydrate* is a chain of carbons with a hydroxyl group (also known as an alcohol group) on the end. A hydroxyl group is made up of an oxygen and a hydrogen atom and is represented as (-OH).

- A *protein* also consists of a chain of carbons. In this case, however, the carbon chain has an amino group—a nitrogen atom and two hydrogen atoms (NH_2)—attached somewhere on the molecule, and an oxygen connected at the end.

- *Lipids,* or fats, dissolve easily in organic solvents but not in water; they are fat soluble. Triglycerides, phospholipids, sphingolipids, sterols, vitamins, and fatty acids are different types of lipids that perform various functions in the body.

- One member of the lipid family, a *fatty acid,* is a chain of carbons, with a carboxyl group at the end. A carboxyl group consists of an oxygen atom bonded to a carbon atom that's also bonded to a hydroxyl, and is represented as (-COOH).

These days, we hear so much about how bad fats are for us, that you may be wondering what beneficial functions they could possibly serve in the body. In fact, without lipids, life as we know it could not exist—indeed, it could not have developed on our primordial earth. To understand the important roles that lipids play in maintaining life, we need to take a step back a few billion years to learn about the very first inhabitants of our planet, algae—plantlike organisms that use carbon dioxide and water to synthesize their own food to survive.

Algae grew abundantly in our primordial seas. In order for algae to extract life-sustaining nutrients from the sea, while still maintaining structural integrity, these organisms had to evolve to suit the environment. Over time, the algae developed a cell membrane to control what went into the cell and what was allowed to pass back out; today, all living cells—animal, fungal, and plant—share this requirement of a cell membrane. Algae also developed a cell wall to act as a skeleton, or framework, to help protect the fragile cell membrane.

Living in the seas, algae were in constant danger of being weakened by excess water absorption. There was fluid inside the cell, and water all around the outside of the cell. Without the cell membrane, water would seep unopposed into the cell and further dilute the cell fluid. The cell membrane had to be constructed in such a way that it would allow specific nutrients to be pulled in from the environment without allowing in excess water. It also had to be able to expel waste products—again without letting water in or losing intracellular constituents.

The secret of the cell membrane is its composition of a specific group of fats, called *structural lipids.* These help repel water and filter in the materials that the cell needs for nutrition. If you have ever seen an oil slick on top of a body of water, you've surely observed that it blocks other materials from getting under it, and that it keeps the water underneath it confined. The cell membrane is designed as a double layer of these lipids to form a protective barrier.

The cell wall provides a structural integrity to the skeleton of the cell, and the cell membrane provides the gateway for the cell's absorption and excretion, that is for transferring chemical substances into or out of the cell. This fat-containing structure is the key to life for algae right up the food chain to all plants and animals.

"GOOD" OXYGEN VERSUS "BAD" OXYGEN: FREE RADICALS

When it comes to our health, the element oxygen is a bit of a double-edged sword. Without oxygen, advanced life could not have developed on this planet. But it also is the source of so-called *oxidative stress.* Oxidative stress produces "molecular thugs" called *free radicals* that can destroy cell membranes.

First, let's review some basic chemistry to understand why this happens. Remember those tiny particles called atoms that we discussed earlier? Each atom has a nucleus, or central core, containing smaller particles known as protons that have a positive electrical charge. Orbiting around the nucleus of the atom are particles called electrons, which are even smaller than protons and have a negative electrical charge. Surely you've heard that "opposites attract." In the case of molecules, opposite charges attract. Molecules, which are built from a combination of atoms, may have a net positive or negative charge depending on their number of protons and electrons, and will therefore attract other atoms or molecules of the opposite charge to neutralize or stabilize their own charge.

A free radical is a highly charged molecule that is missing one electron. Free radicals go banging around in our bodies trying to steal an opposite charge from other unsuspecting organic membranes in order to become stable. This may seem like a silly image, but think of the free radical as a house with only three sides. Such a house is clearly unstable so, in order to stabilize itself, it roams the neighborhood and peels a side off a house down the block. The new three-sided house down the block will soon collapse—unless it now steals a wall from another house, causing a destructive chain reaction. This is what happens at the molecular level. When a free radical steals an electron from another molecule, the host molecule is left unstable. The integrity of the cell is destroyed, and the cell, like the house, will collapse.

Free radicals can be produced by many things, including normal metabolism, disease, stress, tobacco use, and pollution. These nasty molecules attach themselves to cell membranes, destroying their integrity, to acquire the needed electron. In the case of algae, a free radical would attack its surface cell membrane. In the case of humans, it may attack any of our cells' membranes, or even the membrane surrounding a cell's internal mitochondria—the powerhouses within cells that make energy from the food we eat.

When oxygen is used in the cells' energy-producing reactions, the process is called "oxidation." However, spare parts (singlet oxygen, hydroxyls, and peroxides) are generated from these events as byproducts. In order to understand this in terms of the damage these free radicals can do to cell membranes, and thereby, to any tissue or organ, it may be helpful to think of rust, a form of oxidation that we can see any day in any number of places. It is this chemical process of oxidation that literally destroys metal—so imagine what it can do to the body! This is the reason free radicals are also called *oxidants.* And chemicals that counteract their effects are called *antioxidants,* or "free radical scavengers."

If a molecule has at least one double bond (two connections between atoms), it is able to pick up and neutralize a free radical. When a free radical attaches itself to a molecule that contains double bonds, it can successfully connect to one of the bonds to make itself whole, still leaving the host molecule with a single stabilizing bond. The host will not collapse. In this way, a double bond protects cell membranes and renders free radicals harmless. The more double bonds your cells have, the more free radicals you can neutralize. End result? More resistant cell membranes and a healthier body.

DHA has been selected through evolution as a major building block of cell membranes because its molecular structure contains *six* double bonds. Since double bonds, with electrons to spare, are an easy target for free radicals, DHA can act as a biochemical sponge *and each molecule can potentially neutralize up to six free radicals attacking a given cell.* This description is rather simplistic because the loss of double bonds does change the characteristics of the molecule, as I will discuss later.

So this exquisite building block not only provides strength and flexibility to the membrane, but it also has a built-in defense

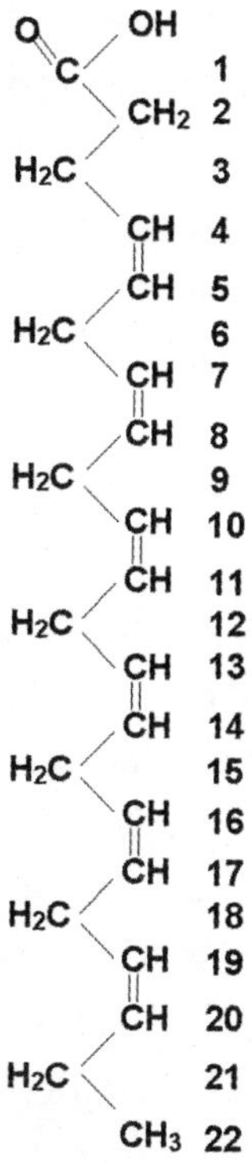

FIGURE 1.1. DHA Molecule Structure.

mechanism to protect the membrane from damage. Figure 1.1 illustrates the structure of the DHA molecule showing its six double bonds (two straight lines between CH molecules).

"GOOD" FATS VERSUS "BAD" FATS

Just as most of us assume that oxygen is always a good thing (until we learn about free radicals), we are also conditioned to think that fat is always as a bad thing—until we learn about omega-3 fatty acids.

I was in high school when I first learned about proteins, fats, and carbohydrates; to this day, I remember my biology teacher stressing that *all* nutrients of these were important parts of metabolism. (Metabolism is the sum of all physical and chemical actions that build, maintain, and transform energy for living organisms.) Even then I found it hard to believe that fats could be vital to metabolism. When I was growing up, "fatty" and "fatso" were derogatory terms directed at kids who were overweight.

I carried the "fat is bad" message with me throughout all my school years. As a pre-med major in college, I took many chemistry classes in which I learned all about the chemical structure of proteins, carbohydrates, and fats. But even as I was learning about different kinds of fats, I still had the notion that all fats were harmful. I learned without understanding and I carried that critical lapse over into medical school.

Unfortunately, medical school did not teach me the importance of what you feed your body's cells and cell membranes. Every medical student was required to take an all-important biochemistry course, but only three hours of the entire course were devoted to nutrition. I believed what I learned was correct information, and I assumed that if there were only three hours of nutrition instruction in all those years of medical school, nutrition itself couldn't be all that important. How wrong I was!

It turns out that my high-school biology teacher was right. Over the years, I have learned that carbohydrates, proteins, and fats do indeed all play important roles in basic metabolism. Proteins are important for genetic development and growth. Carbohydrates are important for immediate energy, as well as energy storage. But I was startled to find that fats are equally important. In fact, fats provide more than twice the energy of protein or carbohydrates. Long-chain fatty acids, called "essential fats," build the brain and the eye's retina (up to 30 percent of the brain and the retina are composed of DHA!), help construct the insides of joints and blood vessels, and contribute to every cell membrane in the body. Yet, even in the face of this evidence, it is difficult to shatter the "fat is bad" myth.

Our society is flooded with advertising images of "ideal" super-thin super-models. And we fall under the spell of the media's anti-fat propaganda. We take "fat-trapping" pills, and metabolism boosters, and try to cut fat as much as possible from our diet. Many of us even buy expensive exercise machines that, in many cases, eventually end up as convenient clothes hangers. In short, we are programmed to do everything we can to avoid fat, but still are attracted to it. So we end up eating cheesecake and drinking diet soda. Sound familiar?

Well, if I am to convince you that some fats can be your "friend," I must first start by defining fatty acid. A *fatty acid* is a straight chain consisting of two to twenty-two carbons with a terminal carboxyl group at the end. It's the carboxyl group at the end that is the "fat soluble" part. Proteins and carbohydrates are not considered fat-soluble.

Figure 1.2 on page 15 shows the basic structure of a saturated fatty acid, such as that contained in butter, margarine, corn oil, or meat. Notice that there are no double bonds between its carbon

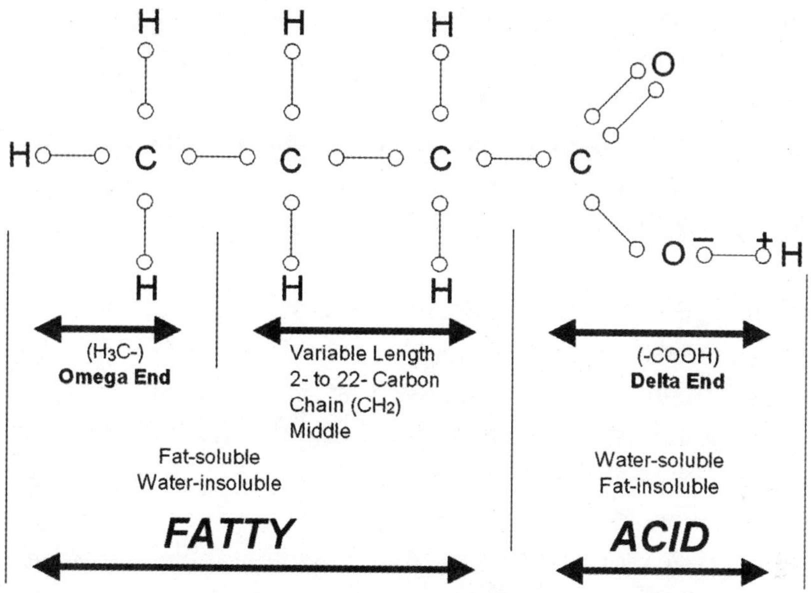

FIGURE 1.2. Basic Fatty Acid.

atoms. Most of us consume an over abundance of these every day. Saturated fats are attracted to each other. They clump together and accumulate in cells and become the fat we all see after the holidays.

THE CHAIN GANG

Fatty acids are classified by the length of their carbon chains. A short-chain fatty acid is made up of four to six carbons, a medium chain fatty acid consists of eight to twelve, and a long-chain fatty acid has fourteen to eighteen. Fatty acids with twenty carbons or more are termed very-long chain fatty acids. The long chain carbons exist only as oils in liquid form. A solid form, such as butter, is composed of short-chain saturated fats. (For the sake of convenience, throughout this book, I will simply use the term "long chain" for the soon-to-be-introduced omega-3 and omega-6 polyunsaturated fatty acids.)

There are two types of fats: *saturated fats* and *unsaturated* fats.

Saturated fats—the so-called "bad" fats—lack double bonds and therefore, while they do supply energy, they do not support cell membrane function and they aren't able to protect us from free radical damage. Saturated fats occur naturally in animal products, and they are also synthetically made, or processed. In either case, the longer-chain fats have been broken down into shorter units that lack double bonds.

The so-called "good" fats are the unsaturated fats, found in seeds, some oils—such as olive oil and flaxseed oil—certain grains, fish, and algae. Unsaturated fats may contain one to six double bonds. *Monounsaturated fatty acids* (MUFAs) have only one available double bond. *Polyunsaturated fatty acids* (PUFAs) have more than one double bond. With multiple double bonds, PUFAs can scavenge more free radicals than any other molecule and add elasticity to the cells.

You may have seen television commercials that boast about how a product is rich in polyunsaturated fats, and is therefore the best product you can buy. Certainly, food products that contain PUFAs are better than those that contain only MUFAs, and indeed better than foods high in saturated fats, but there are different types of PUFAs. It's important to understand that, while all PUFAs are good for you, they are not *equally* good for you. DHA—the "PUFA Supreme"—has six double bonds, making it essential for supporting cell membrane integrity and function.

Polyunsaturated fatty acids are also known as "omega fats," as well as "essential fatty acids" or "essential oils." They are termed *essential* because, while the body requires them, generally speaking, it cannot manufacture them, so it's essential that we get these fats from dietary sources. Essential oils can be designated omega-3, omega-6, or omega-9. "Omega" in the chemical term denotes the beginning of the molecule, and the number denotes the first carbon that has a double bond (i.e., the third, sixth, or ninth). An omega-3 fatty acid is a carbon chain in which the third carbon shares a double bond with the fourth carbon in the chain (see Figure 1.1 on page 13). An omega-6 fatty acid has its first double bond at the sixth and seventh carbons in the chain, and so on.

Artificially produced fats are known as trans-fatty acids or trans-fats. While the molecules of the good PUFAs are arranged in what scientists call the *cis* form—an appearance of smooth bends—trans-fats' molecules are in the shape of staircase steps. No animals can use a trans-form fat for essential functions. These fats are made from processed (hydrogenated) vegetable oil, and are just as bad as the saturated fats found in animal products such as dairy products. You'll see the words "partially hydrogenated vegetable oil" in the ingredients of most of the cookies and chips in the snack aisle, as well as in many other prepared foods. Whether artificially produced or naturally occurring, trans-fats have a tendency to accumulate in the body around linings such as intestinal walls and blood vessels. These are the *bad* fats.

Because it's so important for us to be aware of the different types of fats in our diet, fat content now is listed on the nutritional label of all foods. The fats are broken down into percentages of saturated and unsaturated. The next time you buy a jar of peanut butter, take a moment to look at the label. Most brands contain approximately 30 percent fat, but they vary widely in the percentage of "good" unsaturated fats. Since trans-fats are not yet listed separately on most food labels, you can simply subtract the combined percentages of saturated and unsaturated fats from the total fat to see how much of this truly useless type of fat may be included in a product.

The next chapter will more closely examine the differences between omega-3 and omega-6 fatty acids and their functions in the body, and talk about the benefits of DHA, docosahexaenoic acid. It's a long name, and there's a long list of organs and body systems that require this omega-3 PUFA to function optimally, including your brain and nervous system, the retinas of your eyes, your muscles, and the surrounding membrane of every living cell.

KEY POINTS

- Algae, alone for a billion years, were protected from turbulent seas and noxious gases by their cell membranes.
- Free radicals, also known as oxidants, are highly reactive molecules that need to be neutralized so they can't damage cells. There are water-soluble and fat-soluble anti-oxidants that will scavenge these free radicals. But the cell membrane remains the last bastion of defense for all cells, from algae to your retina.
- Cell membranes are made up of long-chain fatty acids that provide structure, flexibility, and protection for the cells.
- Fats can be unsaturated or saturated, and may be thought of as "good" (healthy) or "bad" (unhealthy). Now's the time to start reading food labels!
- Long-chain polyunsaturated fatty acids are divided into the two most important groups by the location of the first double bond. Omega-3 fatty acids have the first double bond after the third carbon, omega-6 fatty acids have the first double bond after the sixth carbon, and omega-9 fatty acids have the first double bond after the ninth carbon.
- DHA is so important to the contribution of each cell's membrane barrier that 30 percent of the brain and retina are composed of this crucial polyunsaturated fatty acid.

CHAPTER TWO

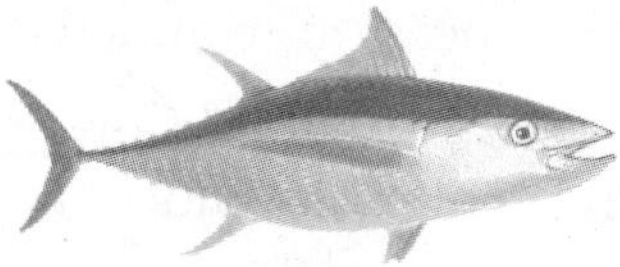

Cell Biochemistry (or Why the Cat Needs the Mouse)

When a good meal comes along, you'd better pounce on it!

—DOC ABEL

Have you ever seen a mouse stalking a cat? Of course not! We all know that mice don't eat cats. Besides the size difference, which would make catching a cat difficult for a mouse, mice don't *need* to eat cats. They need to eat plants and grains. However, most of us have seen a cat stalking a mouse. So have you ever wondered why cats eat plant-eating mammals like mice? Like humans, cats—and all mammals for that matter—need substances that can be found lower in the food chain in plants or plant-eating animals. In watching the cat stalking a mouse, we may wonder at the grace of the cat, or we may simply be glad to be rid of another mouse. But we usually don't think, "Hey, there's a mammal looking for essential fats to enhance his night vision and concentration."

WHAT YOU DON'T USE, YOU LOSE

Fish is another favorite in the cat's diet. If the fish has come from the cold and deep blue sea, it will contain that primo fatty acid: DHA. This important nutrient was once abundant in our own diets. Our early ape-like ancestors wandered down to the coast and ate fish that had grown to an edible size by feeding upon algae—which, not coincidentally, is widely recognized as the best primary source of DHA.

These first humans had no need to manufacture DHA for themselves, since they could simply obtain it from the foods around them, along with other important nutrients. The laws of genetics being what they are, those who employed this simpler method for obtaining DHA were favored. Why? Because manufacturing DHA takes a great deal of energy. So, we advanced along the line of least resistance, getting DHA without our bodies having to exert the energy to manufacture it.

With DHA and other vital nutrients so abundantly available and regularly consumed, the brains of our ancestors developed to what we now know as normal human size and capacity, which over the millennia has given humans a mental advantage over other carnivores. But ironically, because we were able to take advantage of food sources that provided necessary nutrients "ready made," over this same time, any inherent genetic capability our bodies once had to manufacture these nutrients has been lost.

The human brain requires a 1:1 ratio of omega-3 fatty acids and omega-6 fatty acids. So long as we could simply help ourselves to these nutrients, we did not have to worry. But as our society became more industrialized, and processed foods became temptingly convenient, even though DHA has always remained an absolutely critical element for good health, we began to have less and less contact with its primary dietary sources. The omega-6s still are readily available in many of the foods we eat, but it's now much more difficult to fulfill our requirement for omega-3s.

The problem has worsened over the years. Factors such as over-farming, increased population, and our susceptibility to the convenience of (generally unhealthy) fast foods, have altered our diets so that we no longer are getting our most vital nutrients simply by eating whatever we find close at hand. This is most especially true of DHA. And, as mentioned earlier, we cannot biologically "convert" the food we do eat into DHA. As a result, we often find it necessary to take supplements.

SEPARATING THE MEATS FROM THE CHAFF

In Chapter One, I confessed about my troubled past with fats. I preached the "anti-fat" gospel to my patients, until I began to study nutrition—and I mean *really* study nutrition. Studies that were being published regarding cardiovascular disease first triggered my interest. These studies focused on *cholesterol* and *triglycerides* as contributing factors to cardiovascular disease and I wanted to know more. (See Chapter 7 for an in-depth discussion of the connection between triglycerides and heart disease.) As I mentioned, nutrition had not been a big part of my formal education, and I felt a little at sea when it came to understanding the significance of these studies, so I decided to enroll in some nutrition courses at the University of Delaware. These classes not only opened my eyes, but they changed my practice, as well. For example, although I'd read many medical studies reporting that eating fish is heart healthy, it wasn't until I understood the basics of nutrition that I finally understood that fish oil contains beneficial omega-3 fatty acids. More important, I learned that these omega-3s were the "right fats"—the MUFAs and PUFAs we discussed in Chapter 1—that help build and develop the body.

I also learned that grain-fed cattle have more muscle mass, and therefore more meat, than cattle that graze, but they also have white fat. I'm sure you've seen meat displayed at the grocery or the butcher's shop. Most cuts will have a border of fat. While you may be able to trim off the fatty border, you can't trim the white marbling out of the meat. In fact, nearly every chef will tell you it is the marbling that gives the meat that great taste and makes it nice and tender to chew. Well, be that as it may, the white fat is saturated fat, and saturated fat is of limited value to your body. It mainly stores energy in the body for leaner times. But unlike their grain-fed kin, cattle that graze on grass build up *yellow* fat, which is partially *unsaturated* fat—and much better for you.

Likewise, domesticated pigs have up to 80 percent saturated fat compared with less than 20 percent in wild pigs. Wild turkeys have brown breast meat that is loaded with good fats and mitochondria. Domesticated turkeys, however, have white breast meat, which has minimal amounts of good fat; this is why they cannot fly. When applied truthfully, the label "free range" can make a difference in the health benefits of meat products.

Saturated fats are found only in animals and processed foods. Plants contain only unsaturated fats. But it's easy to be fooled. For example, the production of a vegetable oil for cooking requires hydrogenating—or adding hydrogen to—the double bonds of the original PUFA, changing it into a saturated fat to increase its shelf life. So vegetable oils, despite the name, are not real representatives of plant products. Saturated fat and protein may build a bigger body, but they will not help grow a bigger brain, or neutralize free radicals.

THE FACTS ABOUT FLAX

Having said all that, you may be wondering why whole grains like your morning bran flakes are good for you, but grain-fed beef is not. To understand that a little better, we'll have to discuss the facts about flax.

As a very good source of omega-3 fatty acids, flax has been enjoying quite a run on the health-food hit parade in all its forms—supplements, seeds, and pressed oil. Well, omega-3s are all good, but not all omega-3s are equally good. Many people think, "I'm eating flaxseeds, I'm using flax oil, I'm getting my omega-3s. I'm in great shape." Eating flaxseeds is better for you than eating peanuts, corn, or foods with lots of saturated fat. Flax won't hurt you and it will, in fact, do you some good, but it's not the best member of the omega-3 fatty acid family.

Flax oil is a fatty acid composed of eighteen-carbon chains. The most beneficial fatty acids are those very-long-chain essential oils with twenty to twenty-two carbons. The fact is that we are very poor in our ability to use enzymes to build chains longer than eighteen carbons. Conversion from eighteen carbons to twenty-two in a chain simply takes too much energy, especially as we grow older and have less energy to spare. Building or converting carbon chains has a cost: when you take energy and antioxidants from other parts of the body, you're basically detouring them from the other important functions they were already engaged in. If you can, you may as well save that cost, right? That's what our brainy ancestors did when they went straight for the fish.

THE COST OF CONVERSION: OMEGA-3 AND OMEGA-6 PATHWAYS

Eighteen-carbon molecules are the raw materials for two separate pathways that provide structure and messengers for all cells. A *pathway* refers to the direction in which chemical compounds are built from a basic chemical to a more complex compound. The two fats that may be constructed from the eighteen-carbon chain are called *linolenic acid* (LNA) and *linoleic acid* (LA). The names are nearly identical, but there is a world of difference between the two. These two fats are the starting points for what are referred to as the omega-3 and omega-6 biochemical pathways. Your body uses these pathways to convert both LNA and LA into "good" fats. It's important to note that the end point of the omega-3 pathway is DHA—the primary building block of the central nervous system, and a critical component of every cell. Figure 2.1 below details how these paths produce the beneficial omega fats.

Fatty acids in the omega-3 pathway are converted to substances that increase immunity, lower blood pressure, thin the blood, and decrease leakage and swelling in blood vessels. Some of the chemicals that are part of the omega-6 pathway, on the other hand, are converted to hormonelike substances called prostaglandins that can cause inflammation. The omega-6 derived prostaglandins constrict blood vessels and stimulate blood clotting. Inflammation has its place in the body, primarily to kill

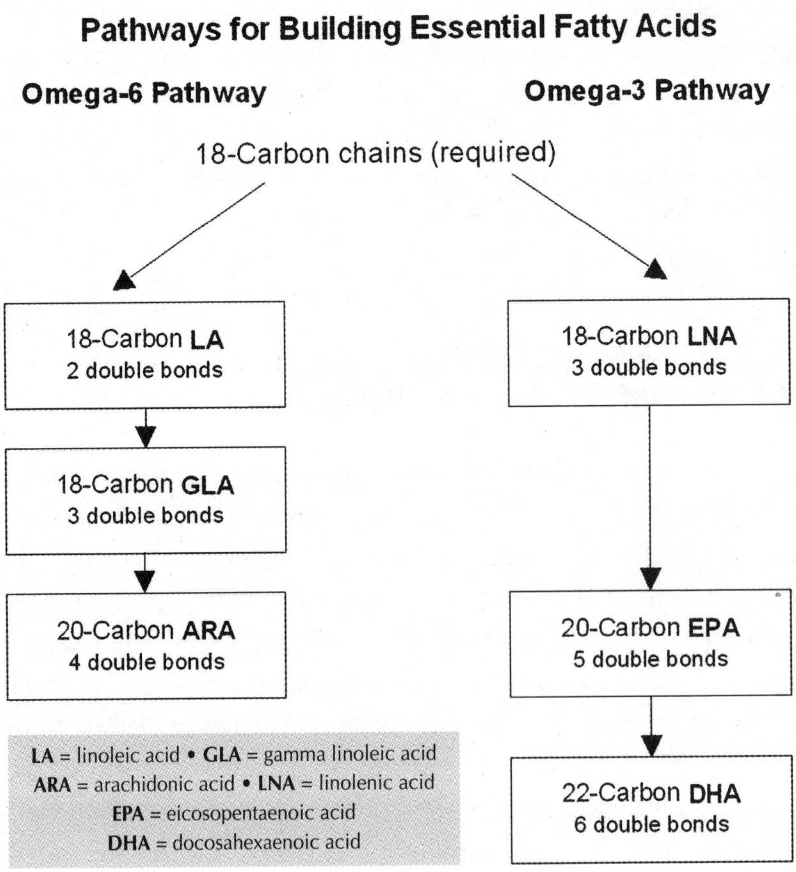

FIGURE 2.1. Pathways for Building Essential Fatty Acids.

aberrant cells, but in most other cases quieting inflammation is preferred to stimulating it. Thus, in the end, we want more of the omega-3 fatty acids—that is, DHA—in our diets to promote general good health, although both are needed.

The mammalian body, including the human body, is able to call on stored materials and enzymes that can create carbon chains up to sixteen carbons in length. We need molecules with at least eighteen carbons just to present us with the possibility of creating the twenty-two-carbon molecules via conversion. But if our bodies lack the enzyme that converts sixteen-carbon chains to eighteen-carbon chains, how do we get enough materials to make a twenty-two-carbon DHA? In order to answer that question, we have to return to a little more biochemistry.

Humans—and other mammals—have to get to that eighteen-carbon molecule from terrestrial sources, either by eating plants or by eating plant-eating animals. However, even when we get the eighteen-carbon molecules by eating plants or the lower animals on the land food chain, we humans have a very limited ability to build these eighteen-carbon acid chains into twenty- and twenty-two-carbon molecules. It is difficult for our bodies to convert LNA acid (which has eighteen carbons) into the *eicosapentaenoic acid* (EPA)—a PUFA with twenty carbon atoms in its backbone—that is required for the body to make DHA, our twenty-two-carbon PUFA. LNA must first be converted to EPA, and *then* to DHA, which is only accomplished at a very dear cost, energetically speaking. Likewise, we have limited ability to convert the eighteen-carbon LA acid into the twenty-carbon *arachadonic acid* (ARA). As noted, through evolution, we lost the enzyme that would give our bodies the ability to make these essential fatty acids because it was metabolically more efficient to hunt and gather the abundant essential foods than it was to build the necessary molecules for ourselves. We used our genetic material for more sophisticated functions, such as the opposable thumb, speech, and learning biochemistry.

While we were busy learning biochemistry, the cat was eating our fish—probably one of the most significant, and least recognized, reasons why cats are noted for their intelligence. And we are not the only ones suffering from a decreasing amount of cold-water fatty fish in our diet. A recent study attributed reproductive problems among the penguins in the Antarctic off of southern Chile to a scarcity of their traditional food, mackerel. Penguins, too, need ample essential oils for health and continued existence. In the vast food web (a term I find more illustrative and accurate than "food chain," which implies a direct line from little bug to big bug to bird to cat to . . . well, you get the picture). Algae and plankton in the sea really are the starting point. They provide long-chain (twenty- and twenty-two-carbon chains) omega-3 fatty acids that are much closer to the final forms used in the brain. Algae are the most prolific producers of essential fats such as DHA on the *entire planet.* Very little conversion is necessary so that all our energy and antioxidants can continue to do other necessary work in the body. Figure 2.2 below illustrates an example of how a common food web works. The mouse eats the grains and uses the eighteen-carbon fatty acids to build the longer-chain fatty acids.

FIGURE 2.2.
An example of a food web.

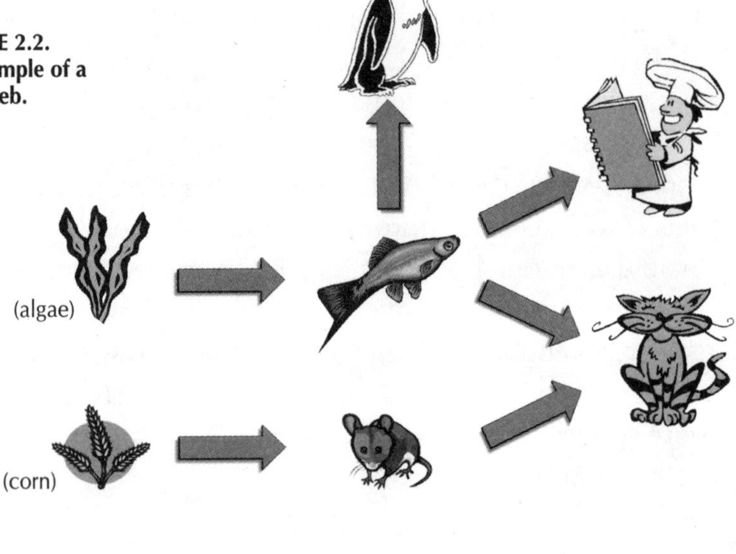

FISH, FLAX, AND THEIR OMEGA-3 FRIENDS

When the cat gets the mouse, he acquires the twenty-two carbon molecules after the mouse has done all the metabolic work for him. But since most of us do not wish to follow a diet rich in mice, I'm going to outline some more appetizing ways you can get these critical supplements in your diet, your body, and your life.

This brings us to the flax. Flaxseed is one of the richest terrestrial sources of the eighteen-carbon structural fats. Only a few seed oils provide a rich supply of LNA. Flaxseed oil is by far the richest source of LNA, but soybean and canola oils are also good sources; keep in mind, however, that soybean and canola oils contain more omega-6 than omega-3 fat. But remember that we are poor converters of LNA up the ladder to EPA and then to DHA.

Fish is an excellent source of LA and LNA, and cold-water fatty fishes that dine on marine algae are rich sources of EPA and DHA. DHA can be found in walnuts, organ meats (liver, for example), some seafood and, of course, algae. You actually could skip the fish part of the food web and get the most DHA directly from marine algae. I'm sure you feel a lot better now knowing that you have the choice between mice and seaweed.

HERBIVORES, CARNIVORES, OMNIVORES, AND THE BRAIN

A lot of our understanding of the importance of fatty acids is very recent. It wasn't until the 1980s that researchers recognized that deficiency of the essential fats caused a failure to thrive in laboratory animals. Restoring essential fats to their diets immediately reversed their condition of poor health. There are many obscure neurologic conditions that have only recently been correlated with disorders of fatty acid metabolism. (See Chapter 6 for a discussion of these disorders.) While the essential fats could be termed "vitamins," because they are necessary to life, our bodies *can* manufacture a small amount from terrestrial plants and grains. Since vitamins by definition cannot be manufactured by the human body, however, the essential fats are not vitamins in the strictest sense.

Vegetarian mammals have to effectively convert vegetable and seed fats into DHA to keep their brain, eyes, and other organs healthy. Animals like mice need DHA, even though some of their vital organs do not need the same ratio of omega-3 to omega-6 fats as humans. It's no surprise, then, that biochemical studies have shown that mice have a very efficient conversion pathway of LNA to DHA. On the other hand, carnivorous mammals can obtain the pre-formed DHA from the meat in their diets—they consume plant-eating animals to get the DHA they need. Unlike mice, the large hunting cats, for example, have such a poor ability to convert LNA to DHA that they cannot survive on a vegetarian diet. They must eat meat and rely on the ability of mice and other animals to make the LNA to DHA conversion for them.

So animals that are herbivores, or vegetarian—deer, hippos, horses, and mice, for example—take in their essential fatty acids from plants and have a greater ability to convert those foods into the molecules that they need for optimum health. By contrast, omnivores must derive their essential fats in varying degrees from plants and meat. Humans are omnivores; we have some ability to convert LNA to DHA, but that ability is not quite up to snuff. We have to take in roughly 30 grams of LNA (found in flax, for example) for our bodies to make just 1 gram of DHA. This is why we need to eat both plants and animals. For us, eating meat is a much more efficient way to obtain the DHA we need.

We have already discussed the direct correlation between DHA consumption and brain size. Interestingly, there also seems to be a correlation between the *way* animals get their DHA and brain size. As mentioned above, mice manufacture DHA to survive; they do not have very large brains relative to body size. African primates, our closest evolutionary relatives, also survive on a vegetarian diet. While they have large bodies, their brains are a smaller percentage of their body weight as compared with humans. There are exceptions, however. For example, baleen whales eat an exclusively vegetarian diet, but have a very large brain. It's important to note, though, that their diet consists of marine algae, or phytoplankton, which are very rich in DHA, unlike terrestrial plants.

It seems that the efficiency of certain biochemical pathways in the body define the requirements for dietary DHA. The mouse may need only the seeds, but the cat needs the mouse. Humans are much more cat-like than mouse-like and, along with dolphins and whales, we are the only animals that require a one-to-one omega-3 to omega-6 ratio. Considering the company we keep, it would appear that DHA contributes to a higher functioning intelligence.

HOLES IN THE WEB

Let's return once more to our cat and mouse. When grain becomes scarce the mouse feeds elsewhere, and the cat goes hungry. This is bad news for the cat! There is an even worse scenario, however. If humans build homes on what was once the mouse's field, the mouse has to change his diet and live off our garbage, which is not rich in grains or essential fatty acids. And when the food web becomes deficient in essential fats, we begin to see the consequences. The cat still gets his meal, but starts to lose his hearing, eyesight, and memory earlier than he should have. Humans have the same deficiency. We dine on processed food and beef, chicken, and pork that has been raised on grains that supply minimal amounts of omega-3 and we are then surprised to find ourselves developing a host of subtle deficiency conditions.

Although no less threatening to our health than other nutritional deficiencies, DHA deficiencies are more difficult to detect. History reminds us that many other nutritional deficiencies remained undiagnosed for a long time. For instance, hundreds of years ago, sailors on long sea voyages would sometimes suffer from scurvy, a condition that causes symptoms such as bleeding gums, loosening of the teeth, and extreme weakness and fatigue. While the symptoms were recognizable, no one at that time understood why they occurred. Then Scottish naval surgeon James Lind made an interesting observation: he discovered that sailors who ate citrus fruits did not suffer the symptoms that their shipmates developed. Today we know that the important nutrient found in citrus fruits is vitamin C, and the scurvy is the classic deficiency disease for vitamin C. Lind developed a method of concentrating and preserving citrus fruit juices for use on extended shipboard voyages, and in 1795, the British Royal Navy began providing a daily ration of lime or lemon juice to all its men. Even to this day, English sailors are called "limeys," because "lime" was the term used at the time for both lemons and limes.

In the nineteenth century, as diets changed yet again, new diseases such as pellagra and beri-beri were identified, but not until many years later did it become clear that these conditions were caused by nutrient deficiencies. In the 1920s, cod liver oil was used to treat rickets, a disease of the skeletal system characterized by soft and distorted bones, resulting from a lack of vitamin D. Doctors found that cod liver oil was very rich in vitamin D, but it took many years to recognize that this fish oil was also rich in omega-3 fatty acids, such as DHA.

"That's great, Doc," you may be thinking, "So now I'm deficient in this DHA stuff. Does that mean my grandmother was right to pour cod liver oil down my throat?"

Well, yes and no. The good news is that cod liver oil is packed full of essential oils and vitamins A and D. These essential oils and vitamins come from the marine algae that cod eat in the ocean. The bad news is that many of the cold-water fish (like cod and salmon) are now being farm raised and they are being fed grain that contains omega-6—the same grains that cows and pigs eat.

Since you already get plenty of omega-6 in your daily diet, the cod liver oil you take today may be no more beneficial than it tastes.

Our current Western diet relies heavily upon hydrogenated vegetable oils, or trans-fats, and contains little cold-water fatty fish. (See Appendix A for a list of cold-water fatty fishes). An insufficient intake of PUFAs has health consequences, including Alzheimer's disease, heart disease, and . . . but I'm getting ahead of myself. Read on, but remember the cat, and hope the mouse had dined well! And, for your own sake, you should hope that the fish have dined well, too.

KEY POINTS

- A brief review of food web shows us that a plant-based diet is richer in essential fats. Without an intermediary element, the human body cannot manufacture a fatty acid carbon chain containing more than sixteen carbons. As a result, humans must take in their nutrient needs through diet.
- Our intake of omega-3 fatty acids—especially DHA—is directly related to the evolution of a larger human brain.
- DHA is not the only valuable long-chain essential fatty acid. Others are necessary for brain development and for the formation of prostaglandins.
- With depletion of our seas and soil, we may not get enough omega-3 fatty acids in order to maintain that necessary 1:1 ratio of omega-3 to omega-6 fatty acids in our brains.
- Man cannot live on bread alone.

CHAPTER THREE

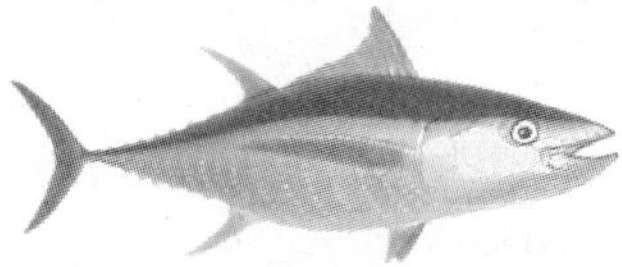

DHA: The Cornerstone of Health

All men may be created equal,
but not all fatty acids are.
—Doc Abel

In the previous chapter, I showed you an illustration of the omega-3 and omega-6 chemical pathways, and then focused on twenty-two-carbon DHA and its six double bonds. Why spotlight DHA and not the other fatty acids? Because all fats are not created equal, and not all omega-3 fatty acids are of equal importance to our health. We have already talked about DHA as being a key component of every cell membrane. In this chapter, I will expand upon that understanding by detailing its importance to maintaining all the different organ systems in our bodies.

AN OMEGA-3 FOR ALL SEASONS

Let's take a moment to consider the leading causes of death in the United States. According to the 2001 preliminary report of the Centers for Disease Control, the fifteen leading causes of death for Americans are as follows:

1. heart disease
2. cancers
3. stroke
4. chronic lower respiratory disease
5. accidents
6. diabetes
7. influenza and pneumonia
8. Alzheimer's disease
9. kidney disease
10. septicemia
11. suicide
12. chronic liver disease/cirrhosis
13. hypertension
14. aspiration pneumonia
15. homicide

I am not listing these common killers to scare you, but rather to give you the big picture of all the different body systems that can be affected by disease. Your heart, lungs, liver, and kidneys are all prone to chronic diseases—and cancer, the silent killer, can strike anywhere in the body. Is DHA the cure for all these ailments, plus the common cold? No. But more often than not it does help.

In 1998, I attended a National Institutes of Health (NIH) symposium. There I learned that cod liver oil, fish oil, and DHA are not all the same; there is a wide variety of fatty acids, including LA, LNA, EPA, and DHA—all those we discussed in the previous

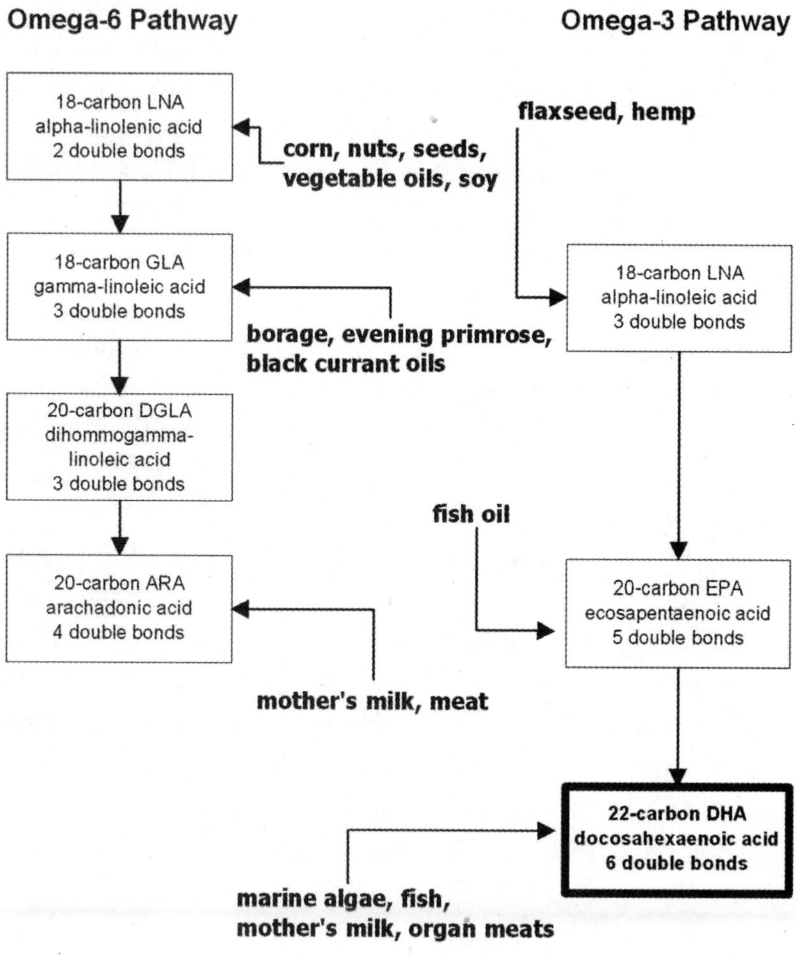

FIGURE 3.1. Essential Fatty Acids and Their Food Sources.

chapter. Figure 3.1 above shows the essential fatty acids and some of their food sources.

I found out that each fatty acid builds on the others and each one has its own purpose in the body. Mostly, though, I finally began to understand the importance of the end-product of the omega-3 pathway—DHA. I was struck by the idea that such a tiny molecule that originated as nothing more than a building block in the cell membrane could also be a crucial building block in every organ system. DHA is not only part of the cell membrane, helping to hold the cell together; it also enhances the function of the cell membrane and plays an important part in the regulation of a cell's cycle—that is, the growth and renewal of the cell. It is essential for cell replication, and there is nothing superior to DHA for the transmission of electrical messages from cell to cell in the body. Also, it facilitates the interpretation of chemical messages—for instance, assisting the function of interferon, a protein produced by cells under attack. DHA makes the cell membrane flexible and resilient. It allows insulin to be more effective on the cell's surface and to stimulate the the influx of blood glucose (sugar) into the cell. Furthermore, DHA probably resists the invasion of foreign proteins like antigens (caused by allergies). Lastly, it forms a matrix for the fat-soluble antioxidants (vitamin A, E, alphalipoic acid, and glutathione synthatase, and so on) to reside. As an integral part of all cell membranes, DHA contributes to the health of all our organ systems. Indeed, the transmission of information and the conduction of nerve impulses that make the heart beat and the mind remember depend on DHA for proper function.

Additionally, recent studies have shown that omega-3 fatty acids may play a role in the function of the immune system. This is notable because DHA is generally associated with central nervous system function and cardiovascular health. DHA is also helpful for such medical conditions as arthritis, depression, heart disease, macular degeneration, and cancer. Omega-3 fats become the sources of certain hormonal compounds called prostaglandins, fatty acid derivatives that serve as chemical messengers to cells and blood vessels in the body. The omega-3 derived prostaglandins, however, suppress inflammation, whereas the omega-6 derivatives increase inflammation, as discussed in Chapter 2.

Table 3.1 on page 37 shows how DHA plays an important role in all parts of your body and how it can lower your risk for certain conditions or diseases.

As you can see, making sure you're taking in adequate amounts of DHA each day through diet or supplementation can enhance your overall body health.

TABLE 3.1. DHA AND YOUR BODY SYSTEMS

Adequate DHA Levels Contribute to	Deficient DHA Levels Contribute to
Normal development of brain and nervous system	Smaller head size, lower IQ, and learning disabilities.
Memory and longevity	Alzheimer's disease, dementia
Normal nerve conduction and signal transmission	Depression, bipolar disorder, schizophrenia, multiple sclerosis, irregular heart rate
Stable cell membranes	Cardiovascular disease, macular degeneration, arthritis, weakened immune system
Increased HDL (good) cholesterol, decreased risk of cardiovascular disease and stroke	Increased LDL (bad) and total cholesterol levels, cardiovascular disease, stroke
Thinner blood	Cardiovascular disease, stroke resulting from thicker blood
Normal blood pressure	Hypertension
Decreased insulin resistance	Diabetes
Healthy skeletal system	Osteoporosis
Normal gastric motility	Irritable bowel syndromes
Normal/Improved mucous production	Cystic fibrosis
Normal eye development and function	Macular degeneration, retinitis pigmentosa
Healthy muscle cells	Decreased muscle tone, lethargy
Reduced inflammation	Increase inflammation due to omega-6 prostaglandins

HOW MUCH IS ENOUGH?

Your diet and your lifespan are intimately related. The diets of the Japanese, the Cretes, many Native Americans, and the Maoris of New Zealand all prominently feature DHA. These peoples consume animals that were fed on DHA-rich plants and grains and therefore live longer and healthier lives. When the Portuguese landed in Mozambique, they discovered eighty- to ninety-year-old people with all their hair and full sets of teeth. It never occurred to them to connect their diet with their longevity. In the 1600s, a European male was fortunate to live to age fifty.

Studies of the lifespans of Eskimos has proven to be very interesting, since a natural assumption would be that they must have a decreased lifespan because the large percentage of fat in their traditional diet. In fact, this is not the case. Although it is true that their diet is at least 60 percent fat, this fat comes mostly from fish and seals, which subsist primarily on marine algae.[1] Eskimos who eat this traditional diet are healthier and tend to reach an older age than other North Americans. Those who have switched to a refined Western diet, however, suffer the same ills as the rest of us.

As you will see in the following chapters, DHA has value in both preventing and treating a wide variety of common medical conditions in people of all ages. Judging from studies that have been conducted to date, it does not appear that there is any upper limit to the amount of DHA one can safely consume; it has not been shown to have any significant negative side effects. One study[2] evaluated students who received 6 grams of DHA a day for three months—100 times their previous daily level—with no noted adverse reactions. Fish oil, on the other hand, is composed of 80 percent eicosapentaenoic acid (EPA), a precursor to DHA, and 20 percent DHA, and can cause some gastric disturbance. Algae is a better source of DHA, since the cell membranes and chloroplasts, or "food factories," of algae contain twice that amount of DHA than is found in fish oil.

So, if you decide to supplement your diet with DHA, just how much should you take? DHA comes in capsule form and should be taken along with a fat-soluble vitamin, such as A or E, and a meal that contains some fat. If you are taking more than 400 or

TABLE 3.2. DR. ABEL'S RECOMMENDED DAILY DOSAGE OF DHA

Group	Amount Daily
Premature infants	40 mg per kg
Full-term infants	20 mg per kg
0–1 year olds	20 mg per kg
1–5 year olds	100 mg
5–10 year olds	200 mg
10–18 year olds	200–400 mg
Pregnant or lactating women	600–1,000 mg
18–50 year olds	600–700 mg
50 + year olds	600–800 mg
Vegetarians	1,000 mg

500 mg per day, I recommend that you take it in divided doses, rather than all at once. Men should consume 4.2 grams of essential fatty acids per day, and women should consume 3.3 grams per day. Pregnant women should double that amount and consume up to 6.6 grams per day of essential fatty acids[3]. Table 3.2 above lists my recommended daily dosages of DHA for people of all ages and walks of life.

My recommendations are higher than previous World Health Organization recommendations because most people do not regularly dine on fish and algae and probably have subtle deficiencies already. Because we have never seen a toxic level of DHA, I am confident that these doses are safe and supportive. The Japanese and Greenland Eskimos eat large amounts of fish and take at least 600 to 800 mg of DHA daily. They usually consume 1,500 to 2,000 mg of DHA and EPA daily with only beneficial effects.[4] See Figure 3.2 on page 40.

Luckily, DHA is an easy supplement to find. Besides the natural sources that I have discussed—cold-water fatty fishes and marine algae, for example—one manufacturer of DHA has been around since research began on this fascinating, and most promising, supplement.

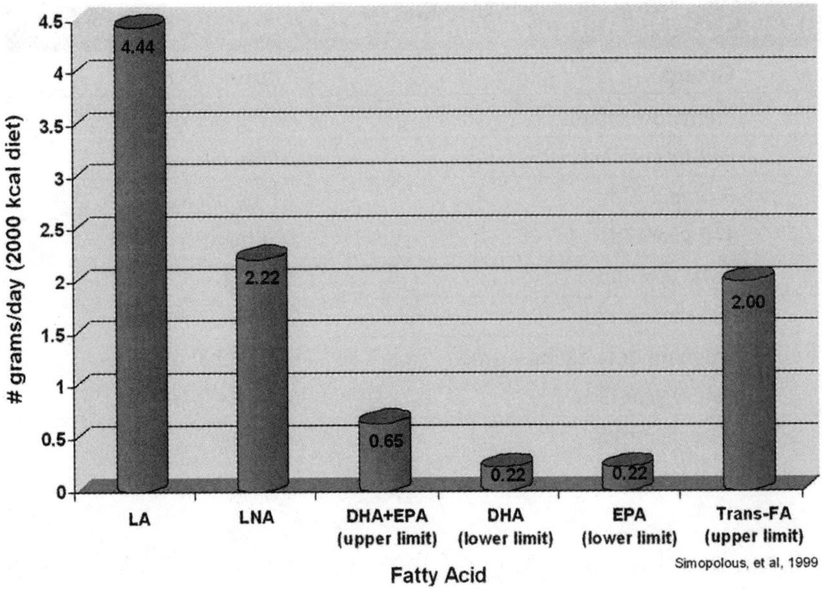

FIGURE 3.2. Adequate Fatty Acid Intake for Adults.

In the 1960s, NASA was concentrating on putting a man on the moon with the Apollo space program. One of the government contractors for the space program was Martin/Marietta, which was developing life support concepts that included placing marine algae in the space capsule with the astronauts. NASA knew the value of having plants in a limited-oxygen environment. Plants—algae, in particular—removed carbon dioxide from the air and replaced it with oxygen. An added benefit was that the astronauts could eat the algae and receive its nutritional benefits.

After the Apollo space program concluded, Lockheed bought Martin/Marietta, and the scientists who were researching marine algae left and started their own company, called Martek Biosciences Corporation. Since the early 1980s, these scientists have studied thousands of species of marine algae to develop the safest, most effective ways of making the benefits of algae available to the general public. Appendix A provides a list of dietary sources of DHA. Appendix B recommends supplemental sources of algae.

KEY POINTS

- DHA contributes to overall body health, and can play a role in reducing the risk of most of the leading causes of death.
- DHA is involved in the structure and function of the central nervous system, heart, joints, and gastrointestinal tract.
- Fish oil, fish, and DHA supplements all contain DHA. Fish oil, however, is 80 percent EPA, and only 20 percent DHA. Algae, because of their cell membranes and chloroplasts, contain 40 percent DHA, making algae a better source of DHA than fish oil.
- Adults should consume at least 3 grams (3,000 mg) of essential fats daily. (See Table 3.2 for specific recommendations for daily DHA intake.)
- NASA has known about the value of DHA for decades, but the knowledge has been slow to spread to the medical community.

CHAPTER FOUR

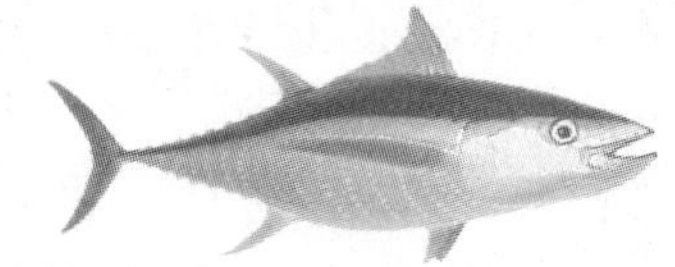

Healthy Mothers, Healthier Babies: DHA and Pregnancy

The infant is at the very top of the food chain, and is the furthest from basic nutrients.

—Doc Abel

If you think back to what we discussed in the previous chapter, you may remember that DHA is usually associated with the central nervous system and that taking DHA is especially important in the growth of the brain and in learning. Well, the most active period for the development of the central nervous system is in utero—that is, while a baby is still growing inside the mother.

During the first trimester of pregnancy, especially the first five weeks, the nervous system and eyes of the fetus begin to develop. Obviously, this is a very critical time and a deficiency of fatty acids during this period can cause a range of very serious problems. Then again, during the last trimester of pregnancy, the brain doubles in size; the fetus is undergoing the "finishing touches" and growing a lot bigger. But did you know that approximately *80 percent* of the growth of the fetus during the final trimester centers on building the brain? Well, it does, and the mother's body is instinctively aware of it. During these last critical months, the mother's body transfers to the fetus the nutrient materials that become the foundations of the baby's brain and nervous system.[1]

The mother's body automatically knows what the best building blocks are, and the mother's placenta selectively pumps DHA and another essential fat, an omega-6 fat called arachidonic acid (ARA), to the fetus from the mother's reserves. DHA and ARA contribute to the nonmyelin membranes (myelin being the insulation material of the peripheral nerves) throughout the baby's central nervous system and to all other organ membranes, as well as to the nerves themselves. As we know, the brain needs a one-to-one ratio of omega-3 fatty acids to omega-6 fatty acids. But since omega-6 fats are so easy to obtain from our daily diets, the omega-3 fats are the most important for us to focus on.

The transfer of DHA to the baby causes the mother's DHA level to decrease.[2] (See Figure 4.1 below.) This is the only time in the human life cycle that the body doesn't retain all the DHA taken in from the diet. Numerous studies have shown that the levels of essential fatty acids in the diet and therefore in the milk of many American mothers is below the recommended amount to support fetal and infant requirements—to say nothing of their own.

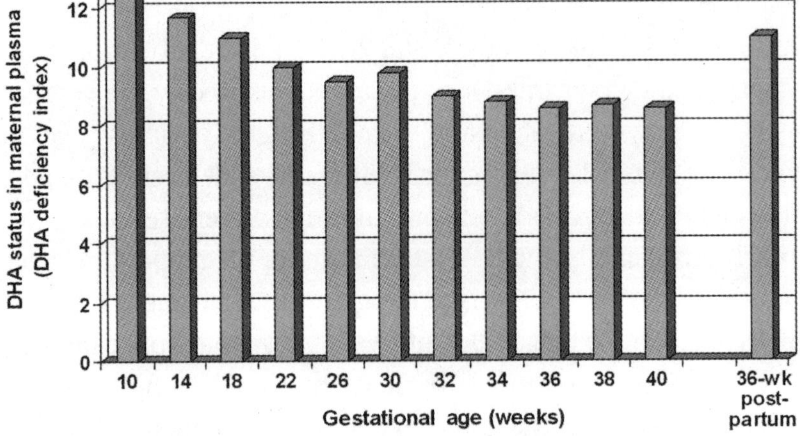

FIGURE 4.1. Pregnancy Depletes DHA from Mothers.

DHA AND POSTPARTUM DEPRESSION

Many of my female patients have told me that during their last months of pregnancy they seem to be more forgetful. I feel certain that this is caused, at least in part, by their personal stores of DHA being depleted as their bodies naturally favor supplying the fetus with all available nutrients. A 2002 Danish study[3] found that women who never ate fish were 3.6 times more likely to deliver prematurely and have underweight infants than women who ate fish once a week.

Once the baby is born, nature still takes care to provide for the brain's growth and development by passing DHA and ARA to the baby through the mother's milk. Unfortunately for the mother, however, this continues to place an additional burden on her reserves. It is likely that the drain on the mother's DHA reserves may be a contributing factor in cases of postpartum depression. This has been borne out in a recent study by Dr. Hibbeln,[4] a psychiatric researcher at the National Institutes of Health. He demonstrated that there is a direct correlation between the DHA levels in a new mother and the incidence of postpartum depression—the lower her DHA level, the more likely a woman is to suffer postpartum depression.

Depression in women is not confined only to the postpartum period; it can show up later in life, too. This may be related to a woman's cumulative intake of DHA throughout her formative years. If a woman does not supplement her diet with DHA or fish oil and has a low level of essential fatty acids when she becomes pregnant, she may be predisposed to a major depression later in life.[5] And if her children are not getting the appropriate supplementation, the trend will continue into the next generation.

FORMULATING MOTHER'S MILK

Research has also shown a connection between a mother's diet and the levels of DHA in her breast milk. Not surprisingly, studies have clearly demonstrated that the amount of DHA in a mother's breast milk is determined by the amount of DHA in her diet.[6] The DHA in the mother's diet is preferentially passed into breast milk and is dose dependent. In other words, the greater the consumption of DHA, the greater the DHA concentration in the breast milk. These levels vary considerably between different cultures. Women in the United States take in very little DHA; in fact, American women rank last in the world in DHA levels.[1]

In the United States, infants are given formula more than in many other countries. These formulas are made to mimic breast milk as closely as possible to provide the baby with adequate nutrition to grow strong and healthy. Great care has been taken to ensure that formulas contain the optimal amounts of vitamins, minerals, carbohydrates, proteins, and fats for the infant. Still, formula is not, as yet, identical to mother's milk, and attempting to ascertain the difference has been the focus of many studies. There have also been numerous other studies that have focused on comparing breast-fed with formula-fed babies at various stages of growth and development.

The differences appear when one compares the long-term achievement, behavior, or performance on IQ tests of individuals who were breast-fed as infants with those who were formula-fed. In a recent analysis, Dr. Anderson[7] of the University of Kentucky established that children who were breast-fed as infants scored on average three to five points higher on IQ tests than children who were formula-fed as infants. A separate study by researchers at Purdue University[8] showed that a group of children who were diagnosed with attention deficit hyperactivity disorder (ADHD) were four times more likely to have been formula-fed as infants than a randomly selected population of otherwise normal children.

To further support the idea that there are differences between breast-fed and formula-fed babies, you can look at the DHA levels of infants. During the first four months of life, a breast-fed baby's blood level of DHA is basically stable. However, the blood DHA level of a formula-fed baby plummets dramatically to barely one half that of the breast-fed baby within four months.[1,9]

Measurements of vision and developmental progression (the progression of growth, orientation, motor skills, and learning during infancy) have indicated that even though formula-fed babies grow bigger more quickly than breast-fed babies, their developmental progression is slowed. In developmental studies, it has been shown that formula-fed babies at ages two to three years old complete an eye chart (with pictures of animals instead of letters) one line higher (larger pictures equal poorer vision), on average, than breast-fed babies at the same age. Clinical studies[1] have now shown that if DHA and ARA are added to standard formulas, the babies' visual development returns to normal, as compared with the vision of the breast-fed infants.

Birch and colleagues[10] demonstrated that infants whose diets are supplemented with DHA and ARA for the first seventeen weeks of life have better visual acuity throughout the first year of life than infants fed standard formulas. Other studies have shown similar results.[11] (See Figure 4.2 below.)

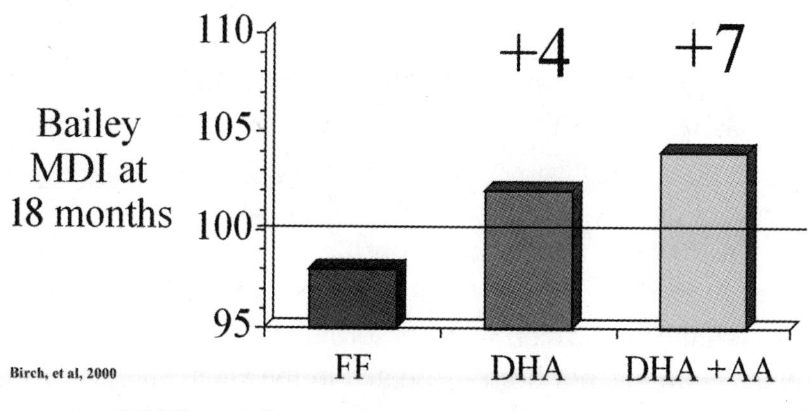

FIGURE 4.2. Bailey Mental Development Index at 18 Months.

DEVELOPMENT AND DHA

Is the slower developmental progression seen in some babies the result of a DHA deficiency? Well, it seems that mothers who play Mozart CDs to enhance their babies' music and mathematical skills would do well to supplement their diets with DHA, as well. As you already know, DHA contributes to overall brain function, especially in early language skills. One study concluded that a sufficient amount of DHA was positively related to babies' abilities to discriminate a non-native language consonant at nine months of age; another showed the same positive relationship between DHA and vocabulary production and comprehension at fourteen months. Another study reported that, at eighteen months of age, the mental development of an infant who was given a DHA/ARA-containing formula was seven points higher on the Bailey Mental Development Index than an infant of the same age fed the standard formulas available in the United States.[11] (See Figure 4.2 on page 47.) Danish researchers associated mental development with the length of breast-feeding in 973 men and women born between 1959 and 1961. Verbal performance and IQ testing was increased with the duration of breast-feeding, being lowest for those breast-fed less than one month and highest for those breast-fed seven months or longer.[12]

Medical evidence supporting the benefits of DHA continues to accumulate. Although breast milk provides nature's best nutrition for a growing infant, the addition of DHA and ARA to infant formulas will at least take these artificial nutrition sources one step closer to that ideal. With the knowledge we have about the benefits of adding DHA and ARA to formula, it is a travesty to have unsupplemented formulas on the market anywhere in the world. At the time of this writing, at least sixty countries have approved the fortification of infant formulas. Yet essential oil supplementation has not been mandated in the United States. As of this writing, one company has added DHA and ARA to its formula. This DHA/ARA addition to infant formulas has reached the highest level of FDA approval. In 2001, Generally Reliable and Safe (GRAS) status for infants and lactating women was granted to Martek Biosciences Corporation for its DHA/ARA product, which is derived from algae. The current consensus is that infant formulas should include 0.35 percent of lipid as DHA and 0.5 percent of lipid as ARA.

While everyone can benefit from DHA supplementation, mothers especially should take advantage of DHA, and supplementation is safe. As indicated in the chart in Chapter 3, the daily recommendation for all women is 3.3 grams of essential fatty acids per day;[13] pregnant women should double that intake to 6.6 grams to make up for the transference of these nutrients to the fetus during pregnancy. And it is essential that at least 20 percent of these essential fats are in the form of DHA.

KEY POINTS

- Breast milk is rich in DHA and ARA, and is an excellent source of the nutrients infants need to grow strong and healthy.
- Breast-fed infants tend to have lower incidences of learning disabilities.
- Research has confirmed that using formulas supplemented with DHA and ARA will improve an infant's IQ and brain development.
- All women of child-bearing age should strongly consider daily supplementation of 600 to 1,000 mg of DHA.
- DHA deficiency results in slower infant development. DHA depletion may result in depression in new mothers and in all of us.

CHAPTER FIVE

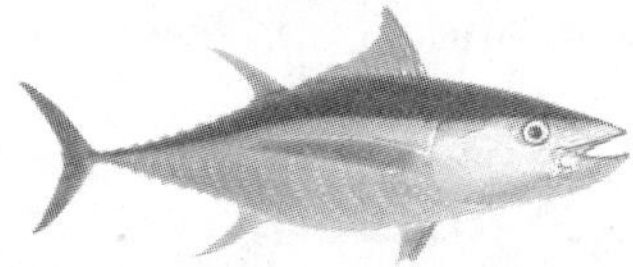

Sight for Sore Eyes

80 percent of our sensory connection to the world is through our eyes.

—DOC ABEL

Vision is one of our most important connections to the world. If your eyes were not functioning correctly you would not only miss a good movie, but you would also not be able to live or work as effectively as you presently do. The simple design of our remarkable sense of sight, which allows us to see the full spectrum of the colors and range of shapes and textures of nature, is truly amazing.

In the simplest terms, the eye is a fluid-filled sphere that contains two lenses called the *cornea* and the *crystalline lens.* These two clear lenses are surrounded and nourished by clear fluids—tears, aqueous humor, and vitreous humor—and are designed to economically focus light and images on the retina, a layer of light-sensitive cells in the eye that carries images to the brain. The sensitive cells that make up the retina are *cones* and *rods,* which have different functions in the eye. Cones transmit color and daylight vision and are tightly packed together in the center of the retina—an area known as the *macula,* which is only 1.5 millimeters in diameter. Rods are located around the edges of the retina and provide night vision and peripheral vision.[1]

FROM LIGHT TO ENERGY TO SIGHT

The incoming light that the rods and cones—collectively called *photoreceptors*—detect is converted to chemical energy that carries nerve impulses to the brain to be translated into the miracle of sight. It takes a great deal of energy for the photoreceptors to convert incoming light to chemical energy. In fact, the receptors in the retina have the highest metabolic rate in the body. For this reason, the blood supply to the retina is critical.

Rods and cones are broken down by the light-conversion process, and must be rapidly restored; the cycle of breakdown and reconstruction is unceasing. When we are in optimal health, the rods and cones are built up again quickly and economically from nutrients produced by the liver and brought to the eyes via our circulation system. Much of this rebuilding takes place at night, when the eyes are closed and the body is relaxed. It should be noted that because this process depends on various body systems working together, a compromised state of health in any one part of the body will adversely affect the efficiency of the whole.

While extensive research has been conducted to fully understand the makeup and function of rods and cones, thus far the most scientific progress has been made on the composition of rods. The outer segments of rods and cones consist of stacks of membranes made up of fatty acids and membrane proteins. Each membrane protein is composed of 60 percent DHA. One of these proteins, the light-activated *rhodopsin,* is dependent in a relative way on the DHA component. That is, the higher the DHA concentration, the higher the rhodopsin density, and the greater the visual sensitivity. The uniqueness of these highly membranous retinal cells is in part due to their high composition of DHA. Since the tightly packed photoreceptors require flexibility and rapid transmission of energy, DHA is the crucial molecule. With its twenty-two carbons and six double bonds, DHA can send 10,000 signals in one twenty-fifth of a second to the deep recesses of the brain for interpretation. There is no computer on the planet that can work that quickly. Figure 5.1 illustrates the structure of a rod with its DHA and phospholipid components.

The importance of the omega-3 DHA composition of the rod outer segment membrane was recently made clear by a study conducted at the National Institutes of Health. Researchers demonstrated that if DHA was replaced with its counterpart from the omega-6 pathway—*docosapentaenoic acid,* or DPA, an omega-6 fatty acid—the membrane structure was disrupted and the rhodopsin energy conversion was dramatically reduced.[2] Clearly then, an omega-3 deficiency can result in vision loss despite ample amounts of omega-6 fatty acids.

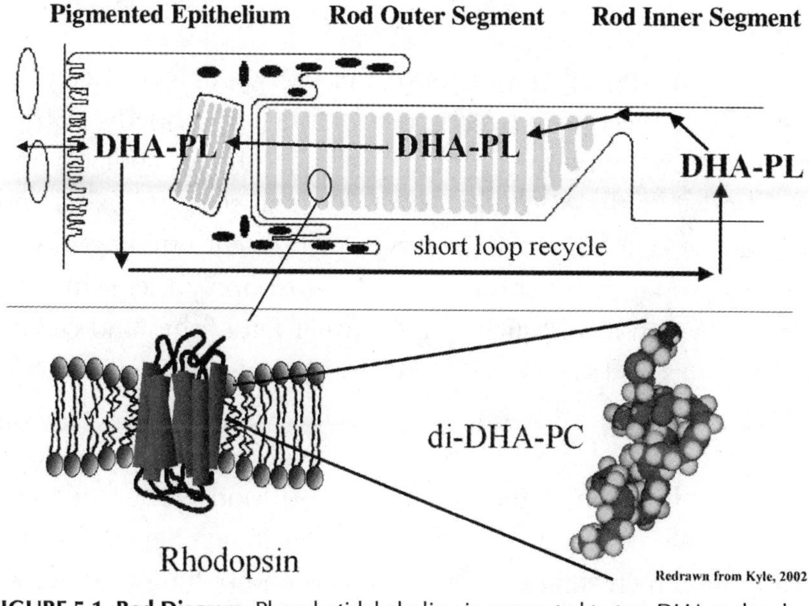

FIGURE 5.1. Rod Diagram. Phosphotidyl choline is connected to two DHA molecules in the rod cell membrane. This combination is called a phospholipid and is a major portion of the lipid bilayer of every cell.

EYE STRESSORS

The eyes are like a car's headlights. You hardly notice they are dimming until either the battery dies or the bulb burns out. The eyes are not only the windows of the soul, but interestingly, they also reflect total body health.[3] Often, we can tell if someone is not feeling well just by looking at his or her eyes. When we are sick, our eyes look tired and dull. But it seems that eye health and illness are connected in some ways that are not highly visible, as well. For example, studies have shown that women with the narrowest retinal arteries face nearly twice the risk of heart disease than do women with normal-sized retinal arteries.[4] This is true even if the individual does not have any other cardiovascular risk factors, such as high blood pressure, diabetes, or family history.

Since the importance of maintaining eye health is inarguable, let's look at the four major stressors to the eyes: poor nutrition, sunlight, unhealthy lifestyle choices, and stress itself.

Poor Nutrition

Just as with the other organs of the body, our eyes need the nutrients supplied by a healthy diet to function properly. DHA is crucial in providing the foundation for good eye condition and total body health. When ultraviolet light and stress (physical and mental) deplete our ocular reserves of nutrient building blocks and antioxidants, we should be able to resupply them through diet. DHA-rich foods, such as cold-water fatty fishes and certain grains, fruits and vegetables can go far in replenishing the necessary components for good health.

What you put in your mouth has a lot to do with how well your eyes function. A diet high in refined foods, food additives, hydrogenated oils, saturated fats, and caffeinated beverages succeeds only in creating more free radicals and putting more stress on your body's reserves. A diet rich in omega-3 fatty acids and antioxidants, along with an adequate intake of water, can neutralize free radicals. What we breathe, drink, and eat helps us maintain the best possible biochemistry and the healthiest eyes.

Water, though not strictly considered a food, should be the most important component of your diet. You should drink six 8-ounce glasses of filtered water a day. Drinks containing caffeine, refined sugars, and artificial sweeteners don't count, because they only add to the body's stress level. Caffeine stimulates urination, so you lose water when you drink caffeinated beverages, and sugars need to be diluted for digestion, so when you excrete sugar or pass it into cells, water goes with it. Artificial sweeteners are considered neurotoxins or excitotoxins—compounds that stimulate nerve endings and are difficult to metabolize—and are finally excreted, taking water with them when they go.

If the antioxidant level in our bodies is depleted, the eyes suffer. It may surprise you to know that the liver is actually key to our vision health because of the important nutrients that are stored there. The eyes draw on these stores to rebuild the rods and cones every night while you sleep. In my thirty years as a practicing ophthalmologist, I have found that the eyes can be the first place that health abnormalities appear if the level of antioxidants in the body becomes too low. These abnormalities, if left unchecked and untreated, in time will manifest themselves in the rest of the body.

Most nutrition experts urge us to eat five to nine servings of fruits and vegetables a day, and most "ordinary people" fall well short of that ideal—at least some of the time. So it's important to make up for the shortage by supplementing wisely. For more information on the value of supplements in general, I recommend a book by Goldberg, Gitomer, and Abel called *The Best Supplements for Your Health*.[5] DHA is an integral part of the retina's rods and cones and is therefore important for normal vision. Other nutrients that nourish these crucial cell membranes include: vitamins C and E, glutathione, taurine, magnesium, zinc, and selenium. Lutein and zeaxanthin are two important carotenoids that are also abundant in a healthy retina. These yellow-colored relatives of the beta-carotene and vitamin A family protect the lens and retina by reflecting damaging ultraviolet and blue light. Lutein also contributes to the macular pigment density (the amount of pigment in the layer just below the retina), which can be evaluated for retinal health. (Loss of pigment will increase the chances of macular degeneration, as I'll discuss later.)

Sunlight

Most of us know to wear sunscreen on our skin when we venture out into the sun, but many of us forget about protecting our eyes. The sun's ultraviolet (UV) rays are very damaging to the eyes. In fact, sunlight is the number one cause of cataracts, and cataracts are the number one cause of blindness around the world. UV rays are also a major risk factor for macular degeneration. Clearly, then, it is important to wear UV-blocking sunglasses. Have your sunglasses checked to make sure they block 100 percent of UV rays.

Unhealthy Lifestyle Choices

Besides eating well and avoiding UV rays when you can, you will really do your eyes a favor by evaluating your lifestyle and taking care to clean up bad habits. If you smoke, now's the time to quit. If you're not exercising regularly, get active. Take stock of your safety habits to make sure you avoid injury at home, work, and play. (Physical injury is stressful—who would disagree?) Moderate alcohol consumption, deep breathing, good sleep, socializing with friends, and positive attitude all help to relax and energize your mind, which is very good for your eyes and the rest of your body.

Another important part of staying healthy is to have your blood sugar levels checked. When blood sugar levels rise, fluid is drawn into the eyeball, which swells the lens and distorts vision. Glucose levels fluctuate depending upon when you had your last meal and what it was. When blood sugar levels drop, eyesight returns to normal. These changes in sugar levels have an effect both at the cellular level and at the organ level. Some cells are unable to remain strong under physical stress and the result of their breakdown may be peripheral nerve disorders, skin changes, kidney problems, and distension of the blood vessels in the retina. Any diabetic knows it is important to exercise strict control over his or her diet in order to lessen the disabling effects of the disease. Maintaining normal blood sugar levels is, in fact, important for all of us, although perhaps to a less obvious degree. After all, abnormal blood sugar levels (high or low) can really cause undue stress on the body.

Cardiovascular and other systemic conditions may also affect vision. As already noted, optimal blood flow to the eyes and brain is critical for processing light to chemical energy and, therefore, to the entire process of sight. If your heart is not pumping properly, your sight might become impaired to some degree. Likewise, if the kidneys are not properly excreting toxins, the important nutrients the eyes depend upon for top functioning can be in short supply.

Many medications, such as common antibiotics and blood pressure medications, are photosensitizers—meaning that they increase sensitivity to light—and, in combination with UV light, they are toxic to the eye. They will speed up the development of cataracts if you do not wear UV-blocking glasses in the sunshine. Check all of your medications and note how your body is adjusting to or reacting to your medications every three months. This minimizes the chance of adverse reactions. Your medical caregivers may decide to reevaluate your need for these medications. Your pharmacist can inform you whether any of these medicines are photosensitizers.

Stress

As you know, stress may be physical or emotional. Our hectic lives, our "bottom-line" mentalities, bad eating habits, poor sleep, and low-grade depression all draw on our antioxidant reserves and starve the eyes of essential nutrients. Like excess alcohol consumption and cigarette smoke, stress hormones, such as cortisol, break down DHA to shorter, more saturated, and therefore less beneficial fats. There is a direct relationship between stress and your body's immune responses, and an adequate level of DHA can affect both. This is true not only for the eyes, but for the entire body. Figure 5.2 below illustrates the relationship between stress, immunity, and DHA.

There are many ways to reduce stress, including yoga, tai chi, acupuncture, visual imagery, exercise, and your chosen form of spiritual practice—just to name a few. Find what works for you. Breathe deeply, meditate, enjoy time with friends, give to others, or change your environment (even moving the furniture around or cleaning the clutter from your home can often be helpful). Relaxation is an important part of the prescription to enhance your health and optimize your vision.

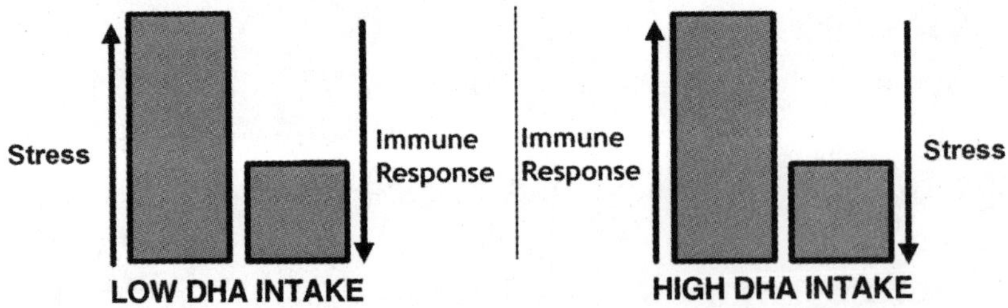

FIGURE 5.2. The Relationship Between Levels of DHA, Immunity, and Stress.

EYE DISEASE

There are numerous risk factors that are common to many eye diseases, including:

- sunlight
- smoking

- low serum lutein
- age
- excess alcohol consumption
- light iris coloring
- injury to the eye
- obesity
- female gender
- incomplete blinking
- family history
- cardiovascular disease
- liver disorders
- diabetes
- high cholesterol
- high blood pressure
- low blood pressure at night
- certain medications, such as steroids, photosensitizers, and statin drugs
- lack of green leafy vegetables and fish in diet
- physical and emotional stress

Eating a healthy diet, protecting yourself against UV rays, reducing stress, and taking steps to lead an overall healthy lifestyle can help you avoid the following eye problems.

Cataracts

The lens of the eye does more than focus light onto the retina—it also protects the back of the eye by absorbing toxic UV wavelengths. The lens is convex, or bows out, on both sides; viewed from the side, it resembles a football. The composition of the lens is high in protein, but over the years this protein denatures, or breaks down. Unlike the retina, which enjoys a rich blood supply, the lens is supplied neither by blood nor by nerves. Consequently, it has to rely on the small trickle of aqueous fluid inside the eyeball to replenish its nutrients and remove built-up waste.

With years of exposure to sunlight, the protein in the lens breaks down and the lens hardens—a process known as photo-oxidation. The lens becomes less flexible and opacities called cataracts form. Cataracts may be central, peripheral, or just beneath the outer capsule, called subcapsular. People who live at higher altitudes or in a "sun belt," need to be especially careful to protect their eyes. Because their eyes are more frequently exposed to stronger light, people who live in these areas have consistently shown a greater incidence of cataracts.[5]

Many people feel that cataracts are an inevitable part of the aging process, but in my experience, this is not the case. Photo-oxidation and early cataracts often may be countered by drinking lots of water and taking in more of the essential nutrients lutein, and vitamins A, E, and C. A study in Australia found that the presence of age-related cataracts was associated with an increased risk of death. That is, participants who had cataracts died sooner than those who did not have cataracts. The presence of cataracts were shown to be a kind of "beacon" indicating other health and life-threatening conditions.[6] What does this mean for you? It means that if you feed your body the right foods, you will decrease your risk of developing cataracts, and quite likely will enjoy a longer life.

Macular Degeneration

The cycle of rebuilding rods and cones in the retina can be derailed by a number of factors, including overexposure to UV light, decreased blood supply to the eyes, poor digestion, and inadequate nutrition. When the fats in the membranes of rods and cones oxidize and break down they form yellowish deposits called *drusen.* Drusen and the loss of pigment beneath the retina are the earliest signs of a condition called age-related macular degeneration (AMD).

Ninety percent of people with AMD have what is known as the "dry" form, while 10 percent have the "wet" or "leaky" form. The dry form is a slow deteriorization that occurs in several stages. The wet form is a sudden leak or hemorrhage from the underlying blood vessels. Fortunately, the dry form progresses slowly, giving those affected time to look for protective remedies. Because the retina has such a high metabolic demand, and because we have so increased our consumption of fast food, we all are becoming candidates for this dreaded disorder.

Smoking, high cholesterol, fair skin, light-colored eyes, and a family history of AMD all increase the risk of this disease. But there is good news: one study has shown people who consume tuna two or more times per week cut their risk of AMD by one-third.[7] Another study reported that 4 or more cups per week of spinach or 6 mg daily of lutein significantly decrease the risk of AMD.[8] Lutein supports the cell membrane, helps reflects UV light, serves as an antioxidant, and also increases the amount of pigment beneath the retina. Lutein is the carotinoid found in the highest level in the eye; other members of the carotinoid family are vitamin A, beta carotene, and lycopene. The same study also showed that older adults who have high blood lutein levels have the same visual acuity as younger people.

There are precautions we can take to prevent and manage macular degeneration. In addition to DHA consumption, researchers have indicated that vitamins A and E, lutein (such as the Floraglo brand, found in many multivitamins), lycopene, cysteine, and the amino acid taurine, along with the minerals zinc, magnesium, and selenium, all support retina health.

A Wisconsin study[7] with participants of northern European

ancestry found that an increased intake of cold-water fatty fish was also related to a reduction in the incidence of macular degeneration. A high intake of saturated fat, on the other hand, correlated with an increase in the incidence of macular degeneration. There is also evidence that high intake of trans-fats is related to an even greater risk of retinal degeneration.

Glaucoma

Glaucoma is not a single disease; rather, it is a group of conditions that affect the optic nerve, the part of the eye that passes signals to the visual centers of the brain. Between 2 and 4 percent of American adults have glaucoma, and may not even know it. The most common form is primary open-angle glaucoma, which is characterized by the fluctuation of intraocular pressure (pressure within the eye, loss of peripheral vision, and changes in the optic nerve. African Americans, Hispanics, and the elderly of all races have higher rates of open angle glaucoma.

Glaucoma is often called the thief of sight because most patients with glaucoma have no apparent symptoms at first. Susceptible people may lose vision at nighttime because their blood pressure decreases and the pressure inside the eye may exert a greater force on the small blood vessels nourishing the optic nerve. This occurs because the medication to treat high blood pressure, which was measured during the day, will be more effective when someone is lying down and relaxed. My recommendation is to take blood pressure medication that lasts only sixteen to eighteen hours. Attention needs to be directed not only to managing intraocular pressure, but to managing blood pressure and overall body health, as well.

Part of the problem with taking medication for high blood pressure is that it causes low blood pressure at night. That is often the time the intraocular pressure is highest, and the combination of high pressure in the eye and low blood pressure can damage delicate nerve fibers. Therefore, patients with hypertension should have their blood pressure checked while they are lying down, and should review with their doctor whether it is advisable for them to take blood pressure medication at night.

Important nutrients for preventing glaucoma include multivitamins, omega-3 fatty acids (DHA especially), sublingual B_{12}, and alpha lipoic acid. Because glaucoma is not only a disease of eye pressure but also one of blood flow to the eye, herbs such as ginkgo biloba or salvia miltiorrhiza, which improve circulation, may help as well. The herbs trifola and coleus forskohlii may also be helpful because they induce physiological relaxation.[9] Certainly, breaking a smoking habit, achieving optimal weight for your height and bone structure, and exercising regularly will also help the management of glaucoma.

Would you be surprised to learn that some of the latest eye drops for glaucoma therapy are derivatives of omega-3 fatty acids? Prostaglandin-like medications—Xalatan, Lumigan, and Travatan—are chemically related to EPA. They work to treat glaucoma by increasing the outflow of fluid. Rescula is a synthetic docosanoid derived from DHA that lubricates the outflow drainage channels.

Diabetes Complications

Diabetes is not specifically an eye disease, but nonetheless, people with diabetes are more susceptible to retinal blood vessel changes, or *retinopathy*, and they also have a higher incidence of cataracts. Fluctuations between high and low blood sugar levels cause weakening of blood vessels and subsequent leakage of blood products into the retina. Sometimes this leakage causes hemorrhages, exudates, or swelling of the macula. Other times new, fragile blood vessels will form, which can bleed into the retina or vitreous fluids.

Increased blood sugar causes excess sugar to accumulate in the lens. The lens then absorbs more water, resulting in fluctuations in vision, as earlier described. Once blood sugar returns to normal, the vision also returns to normal. Additionally, excess sugar trapped in the lens is converted by the enzyme *aldose reductase* into an alcohol compound, which is a contributing factor in the formation of cataracts. Maintaining a normal blood sugar level through dietary choices should be a significant element of everyone's lifestyle.

DHA acts against diabetes in four distinct ways:

1. It is a strong inhibitor of aldose reductase.
2. It smoothes the internal lining of blood vessels.
3. It reduces platelet clotting.
4. It reduces insulin resistance at the cellular level by improving the responsiveness of the cell membrane receptor for insulin.

Vitamin C builds collagen and strong blood vessels and is another especially important nutrient for people with diabetes. Adding vitamin C and *quercetin,* a bioflavinoid with antihistaminic properties, to your diet can be very helpful in the long run. Adding the appropriate supplements to your diet before retinopathy takes place can help fight diabetes-related complications to the eyes.

Dry Eyes

Most of us, at some time or another, have experienced dryness and irritation in our eyes from too much work, not enough sleep, or reading too much. Well, while I have your attention, take a break and blink—*now.*

Fifty percent of people older than fifty years of age have frequent dry eyes because they are dehydrated. Overall dehydration causes drying of the surface tissues of the eye, which include the cornea and *conjunctiva,* a gossamer thin membrane that covers the white of the eye, as well as the inner eyelid. Staring, incomplete blinking, and taking medications such as diuretics, antihistamines, and antidepressants, contribute to the lack of moisture in the tear film.

Our eyes are so enriched with nerves and blood vessels that we immediately realize when a foreign body of any kind enters them—from an elbow to an eyelash. They become irritated and need to be immersed in water. Drinking at least six 8-ounce glasses of water a day rather than drinking coffee and sugary soft drinks will help keep your body hydrated and your eyes comfortable.

A fairly well-kept secret is that the same fats that support cell membranes, primarily DHA, are extremely helpful for people who suffer from dry eyes. Much like an oil slick prevents evaporation of water, the lipid secretions from the *meibomian glands,* located in the eyelids, prevent evaporation of our tears. Every time you blink, tears are forced into the exit ducts. Every time you stare without blinking, there is evaporation. During the winter, the dry heat indoors also increases evaporation of the tears, leaving a more viscous, irritating tear film that does not completely protect the cornea.

Sometimes dry eyes can be symptoms of a more serious condition. For example, the symptoms of a disorder called Sjögren's syndrome include dry eyes and mouth, along with arthritis. DHA has been proven helpful in the treatment of each of the components of Sjögren's syndrome.

My suggestion to counteract dry eyes is to take 500 to 800 mg of DHA daily, in divided doses with meals, and a fat-soluble vitamin. Again, it's also very important to drink six 8-ounce glasses of water every day to keep your body well hydrated. Other measures include taking frequent breaks from the computer, blinking often, and buying a humidifier for your home or office. Occasionally, you may want to use minimally preserved or preservative-free artificial tears if necessary.

Options for resistant cases of dry eyes include punctual plugs, insertable silicone pellets like microscopic champagne corks. With every blink, tears from the eyes drain into the nose. By plugging the aperture of those canals, you conserve the tears you make. Lacriserts are small pellets of a dissolvable lubricant that, when placed inside the eyelid, dissolve slowly and steadily; they will wet the eye for sixteen to eighteen hours. Saligan, an oral prescription medication that stimulates tearing and salivation, is another option. I suggest taking 5 mg twice daily with meals.

Phosphotidyl choline is a constituent of the cell membrane lipid bilayer. As seen in Figure 5.1 on page 53, phosphotidyl choline is connected to two DHA molecules in the rod cell membrane. This combination is called a phospholipid and is a major portion of the lipid bilayer of every cell. One company makes an FDA-approved contact lens called Proclear that includes phosphotidyl choline, which in this case enables the contact lens to bind to water. Additionally, the 62-percent water content of the lens makes it comfortable for marginal dry eye patients.

Retinitis Pigmentosa

Retinitis Pigmentosa is caused by a progressive loss of retinal photoreceptors starting with the rods located on the outside of the retina. There are three different types of retinitis pigmentosa; all have a common appearance but different courses. Loss of night vision is the first sign that the rods are giving out. Eventually the cones may become involved. Scattered pigment splotches and a waxy appearance to the optic nerve confirm the diagnosis. In the most severe form, total blindness can occur, if the condition is left untreated.

While light is damaging to the eyes, it is not the cause of retinitis pigmentosa. The true cause appears to be a genetic deficiency of a certain enzyme (or enzymes) necessary for rebuilding the photoreceptors. Although there is no cure for this degenerative condition, recent research has indicated that there are ways to stop the progression, so people with a family history should seek genetic counseling. For instance, numerous studies indicate a deficiency of omega-3 fatty acids in inherited forms of retinal degeneration.[10] In addition, some recent definitive studies[11,12] indicate that both lutein and DHA, which protect cell membranes in different ways, may halt the progression of retinitis pigmentosa.

Incorporating what we know about the treatment of retinitis pigmentosa, my recommendation is to wear amber-colored glasses outdoors Amber-colored glasses are more effective at blocking blue light rays, as well as UV light. These short wavelengths of light are those that are most dangerous. I also suggest taking digestive enzymes (to more completely break down fats in the diet), multiple vitamins and minerals, and 10 to 20 mg of lutein and 1,000 mg of DHA daily.

Optic Neuritis

There are two types of optic neuritis: inflammatory optic neuritis and vascular optic neuritis. Inflammatory optic neuritis is poorly understood. Of the people who develop the condition, 20 to 40 percent will present initially with multiple sclerosis (MS) or develop it later. The symptoms of optic neuritis include blurred and reduced central vision, loss of color discrimination, and an abnormally sluggish pupil, associated with swelling of the optic nerve.

Multiple Sclerosis is more likely to occur in women who have had multiple pregnancies; in adults 20 to 50 years of age; and in thin, nervous individuals. People who develop MS report repeated episodes of numbness or weakness in various parts of the body. Doctors have found that the eye findings (signs of optic neuritis) and magnetic resonance imaging (MRI) results can confirm a diagnosis of MS.

The other form of optic neuritis is vascular and is caused by the sudden interruption of blood flow to the eye, which causes sudden, usually irreversible loss of vision. This form is more difficult to treat than the inflammatory type. Good cardiovascular health is important in the prevention of this disorder.

DHA is essential to the development and maintenance of the eye and nervous system. The fact that we deplete our essential fatty acid stores of it over our lifetime may allow a variety of degenerative or inflammatory conditions to develop. Multiple pregnancies tend to deplete DHA and omega-3 stores, and fat-restricted diets are low in DHA.

Night Blindness

Night blindness is a condition that develops gradually, in which the individual will either lose his or her ability to adapt to the dark, or not see well at nighttime because of a disturbance in rod cell function. Remember, rods are the photoreceptors that are responsible for enabling us to see at night. Many times, night blindness represents dietary deficiencies that may be immediately improved or reversed with one or several of the following supplements: DHA, vitamin A, lutein, bilberry, or zinc.

KEY POINTS

- The eye is the window to your picture of overall health.
- Many eye problems may be symptoms of a more serious disorder. Because the eye depends on the rest of the body to supply its nutrition, better overall nutrition may be the cure.
- DHA is the cornerstone in the development and maintenance of eye health. It supports cell membranes in the lens, retinal receptors, nerve fibers, conjunctiva, and retinal blood vessels.
- DHA transmits light signals faster than a computer.
- It is crucial to fight omega-3 fat loss with omega-3 fat supplementation in the diet. Clinical trials are now evaluating DHA supplementation in macular degeneration and retinitis pigmentosa.

- If your eyesight is failing, don't assume that nothing can be done. Look for solutions and eliminate the stressors in your life.

- Including DHA-rich foods and supplements in your diet will pay dividends not only for eye health but total body health. Include DHA in your health regimen, and remember to have your eyes examined regularly.

CHAPTER SIX

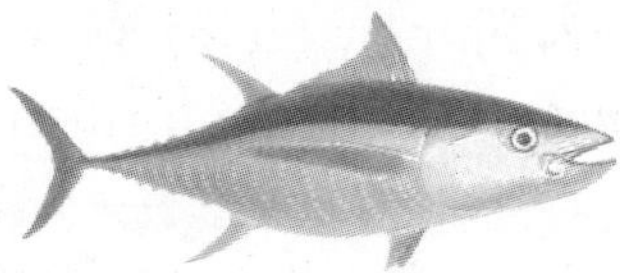

The Brain and Neurologic Heath

Sixty percent of the normal adult brain is composed of structural lipid, i.e., fat.

—DOC ABEL

Dr. Frankenstein used lightning to activate his creature's brain. Fortunately, you don't have to go to such extremes.

Psychiatrists Sigmund Freud and Carl Jung ushered in the twentieth century with their views of the unconscious mind. After some time, psychiatry became a recognized branch of medicine and, for the first time, doctors began to see the possible connections between the mind and the body. It has taken us almost 100 years to understand that the psyche and the neurological system—the mental and the physical, respectively—are intimately intertwined, and can be affected by where we live, what we do, and what we eat. But, in the last 20 years, there has been a flurry of research about the brain and its immense capacities, including mind over body effects.

The brain is like a complex electronic control panel that completely regulates, monitors, and directs the activities of the body. It is an incredibly complex organ with a wiring diagram that we still do not fully understand. There are an estimated 100 billion nerve cells, or *neurons,* contained within the brain, with 100 trillion connections, all of which require chemical messengers called *neurotransmitters* to carry information from one nerve cell to another.

While much remains to be discovered about the brain, we now know that the "wires" of the brain—the neurons—and the "switches" of the brain—the gaps between neurons called synaptic junctions—require a concentrated amount of DHA to function optimally. If you are not getting enough DHA, you may be putting yourself at risk for some of the most common neurologic disorders that we see in America today. These ailments include depression, aggression, attention deficit hyperactivity disorder (ADHD), schizophrenia, Parkinson's disease, multiple sclerosis, and Alzheimer's disease—and they all appear to be linked to the low level of DHA and other essential fatty acids that we take in through our diet. Within two generations, our entire fish-shunning nation could become dyslexic. Both our logic and intuitive systems would be affected. Memory would be shortened or lost, along with tempers, and people would easily rise to anger, perhaps without even being able to remember what it was that got them so mad! To forestall this entirely possible—though highly undesirable—outcome we need to make a conscious effort to increase our DHA intake. Eating liver, walnuts, and algae, or taking DHA or fish-oil supplements all are good ways to make this happen.

FAT AND THE BRAIN

In previous chapters you learned about the development of the infant's brain in the mother's womb, and the importance of maintaining healthy vision throughout life. Now we'll examine the relationship of fatty acids to cognitive function, motor and sensory skills, and emotional health. Although the body and reproductive systems can survive on omega-6 fatty acids, the brain and central nervous system rely heavily on DHA and ARA. Because of its indispensability in cell structure, and its effectiveness at conducting electrical signals, DHA is crucial to proper brain functioning.

In their book *Nutrition and Evolution* (Keats, 1995), Crawford and Marsh describe one study that examined the muscles, livers, and brains of forty-two different mammal species. Although a diverse variety of fatty acids were found in the muscle and liver tissue, all these animals have the *same* fatty acids—the omega-3s and omega-6s—in the brain, albeit in different ratios.[1]

The brain is the only part of the human body that uses one omega-3 molecule for every omega-6 molecule. You must have enough of each if your brain is to function optimally. Taking a lot of omega-6 without replenishing omega-3 disrupts the ratio of the essential fats in the brain, which can result in loss, or dissipation, of nerve function. This happens acutely in women with postpartum depression, but also gradually in people with retinitis pigmentosa, chronic depression, and even bipolar disease. Since turnover in DHA happens much more rapidly than most people realize, bodily functions that you take for granted, like sight, memory and emotional control, could easily short out without warning—just like a blown light bulb.

The brain is composed of numerous complex, interconnected systems that control the musculoskeletal system, all the other organs, and each and every thought. Fatty acids are a part of each cell membrane, as well as the membrane's long tendrils, called *dendrites.* The lipid bilayer of each cell membrane is made up of phosphotidyl choline and essential fatty acids, primarily DHA. Synaptic junctions between cells also contain DHA. The fact that saturated fats are components of the myelin covering and that highly unsaturated fats are used in the signaling structures again points to the role played by DHA in the evolution of the human brain's size, structure, and function.

NEUROLOGIC DISEASES

I will briefly discuss several common neurologic diseases, but as I do, please bear in mind that other disorders may mimic many of these. These may include tumor, infection, vascular disease/ stroke, multiple sclerosis, B_{12} deficiency, and muscle diseases. I cannot overstate the importance of consulting a competent neurologist who can perform the necessary diagnostic test(s) and provide options for treatment, should you experience any of the symptoms described below.

Depression

Over the past 11,000 years, we have cultivated grain as our food staple, but in the most recent 100 years, with reliance upon corn, soy, and hydrogenated oils, we have experienced a marked change in the quality of our "good" fat intake—for the worse. We now consume more omega-6 fatty acids and fewer omega-3 fatty acids.

A worldwide study compared fish intake among different cultural populations and the incidence of major depression episodes. Although this was not a controlled study, the results indicated that lower fish consumption contributes to lower omega-3 intake and, as a result, a higher incidence of depression. (See Figure 6.1 on page 75.)[2] This study also found a correlation between omega-3 intake and developmental changes in the nervous system, as well as changes in perception, IQ, vision, and problem-solving competence. This certainly makes sense when it comes to mood, in particular. Sufficient levels of the neurotransmitter serotonin in the brain help bring mood into balance. DHA is necessary to facilitate the flow of serotonin across the synaptic junction. Plus, higher levels of DHA and ARA in cerebrospinal fluid—the fluid that nourishes and cushions the brain and spinal cord—correlate with higher levels of serotonin metabolites. Conversely, deficiency of DHA in the brain, especially in the area of synapses, seems to relate to low serotonin levels,[3] which, in turn, can lead to depres-

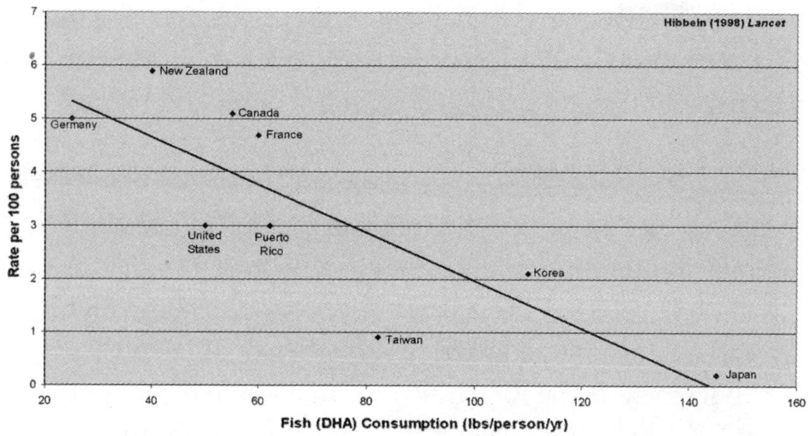

FIGURE 6.1. DHA Consumption Predicts Prevalence of Major Depression.

sion. It makes sense, then, that eating fish on a regular basis is associated with fewer episodes of depression.

When we find ourselves in a stressful situation, the adrenal glands, which sit atop the kidneys, release a hormone called cortisol. This hormone is meant to be a short-lived response that enables the body to deal with an acute stressful situation by increasing alertness, pulse, blood pressure, and response time. Unfortunately, depending upon one's health and lifestyle, stress may not be short lived at all. The long-term effects of chronic physical or emotional stress on the brain are fatigue and depression. Based upon all that we know about the role played by DHA in maintaining optimal mental health, including the studies on postpartum depression cited in Chapter 4, it is very likely that low levels of DHA are at least partially to blame for the body's inability to balance itself in instances of sustained physical stress.

There are many other contributors to depression, which should not be overlooked. They include medications; degenerative conditions such as heart disease, arthritis, chronic back pain, and liver disease; elevated cholesterol; a diet high in sugar; unsatisfactory relationships; and excess alcohol intake. Of these contributors, alcohol is an oxidant, like free radicals, that breaks down polyunsaturated fats (PUFAs) or essential fatty acids (EFAs). Alcohol-treated cats demonstrated a 17 percent decrease in DHA in the brain and an increase in unsaturated fat in both the brain and retina.[4]

Hostility and Aggression

It's difficult not to notice the increase in violent behavior and road rage in our communities. Can this be linked to diet, as well as to lifestyle choices? The answer is yes. Studies show that hostility and aggression are linked to a deficiency of DHA.[2] It's possible that such behavior could be ameliorated by increasing dietary DHA, which would accumulate in the cerebrospinal fluid in the brain. Obviously, there are other contributing factors and predispositions that determine whether a relatively DHA-deficient individual will be depressed and withdrawn or aggressive and hostile. But it should be noted that a DHA deficiency early in life has repeatedly been connected to long-term behavior problems.

Multiple Sclerosis

Multiple sclerosis (MS) is a degenerative disease of the brain and peripheral nervous system, with characteristic acute attacks of focal episodes that may recur and lead to permanent sensory and motor disability. MS is considered a "demylinating disease" because it causes a gradual destruction of the myelin sheath that covers and insulates nerve cells.

At least 350,000 cases of MS are diagnosed annually in the United States and there are four times that number of suspected cases.[5] There is a higher incidence in northern climates, where typically there is more saturated fat in the diet. Infectious agents, such as chlamydia and candida species, have been implicated, but these can be the result of an overactive and misdirected immune system, rather than causes.

Progressive demylenization is generally believed to be irreversible, but the introduction of DHA into the diet has shown gradual improvement as measured by magenetic resonance imaging (MRI) for some individuals in my experience. A decrease in frequency of relapses and improvement in symptoms of MS has been realized with treatment with dietary DHA.[6] It's important to remember, of course, that grains like flax provide only LNA, whereas algae-eating fish provide the longer-chain EPA and DHA. Diets that include excess amounts of animal fats, dairy products, and alcohol increase the levels of the prostaglandin 2 family, which is associated with a higher risk of MS and increase in the severity of symptoms. By contrast, diets rich in vegetables, nuts, and fish increase the prostaglandin 1 and 3 families, which reduce inflammation and improve MS symptoms.

I have found DHA to be very helpful in stabilizing and even improving the health of many of my patients. Alan Tillotson, Ph.D., an herbalist, has created a formula known as the Myelin Sheath Support Formula(tm) that, when used in conjunction with DHA, is extremely beneficial for people with MS.[7] Omega-6 fatty acids have also been listed as being of possible benefit. These include evening primrose oil, borage oil, and black current oil, all of which contain the omega-6 gamma linoleic acid.

There are numerous other natural treatments that can help to manage the signs and symptoms of MS, including vitamin E, alpha lipoic acid, N-acetyl cysteine, B-complex vitamins and B_{12}, phosphatidylserine, coenzyme Q_{10}, vitamin D, and ginkgo biloba or salvia miltiorrhiza—herbs that increase blood flow to the head and neck.

Treating chlamydia and candida, opportunistic infections, has been effective in improving symptoms in some individuals. Also treating attendant stress, anorexia, and dietary deficiencies are important in building up a positive antioxidant balance.

Learning Disabilities

Attention deficit hyperactivity disorder (ADHD) affects an estimated 5 percent of the juvenile population; of this number, more boys than girls are affected. The disorder is generally characterized by inattention, impulsiveness, and hyperactivity, although the severity of the symptoms vary among individuals. People with ADHD may find it difficult to complete their work, and they may avoid tasks that require prolonged concentration because they are easily distracted.

As discussed in Chapter 4, ADHD is less often seen in infants who were breast-fed or given supplements of DHA. Dr. Mary Ann Block, author of *No More Ritalin: Treating ADHD Without Drugs,* is a mother of an inattentive child who had to find her own pathway to success in the management of this disorder. In her book, she cites many studies of the reduced risk of ADHD in the children of mothers who breastfed.[8] Researchers have determined that there is an abnormality in fat metabolism in boys with ADHD; these youngsters have low blood levels of DHA and EPA.[9]

Because the child with ADHD does not understand what is causing the educational and psychological disturbance, punishment is an ineffective response. Pharmaceutical therapy is not uniformly effective and often creates greater internal disturbance—more stress—in many youngsters. Psycho-education is the mainstay of therapy for these conditions. Teaching the person with ADHD methods of organization, time management, and even meditation has been reported to be effective. Additionally, nutritionists and pediatricians are learning to treat the disorder not only with medication, but with changes in diet—for example, advising the avoidance of dietary stimulants, such as sugar and artificial coloring—and the addition of natural supplements.

Dyslexia is a learning disability characterized by an incomplete cycle of information that is now estimated to affect up to 10 percent of the U.S. population, with 4 percent severely affected. Some people with dyslexia also have ADHD.

In the highly regarded British medical journal *Lancet,* researchers reported that five patients with dyslexia who received 480 mg of DHA for one month showed significant improvement in reading ability and behavior when compared with untreated participants.[10] Not all studies indicate that DHA or a mixture of essential fatty acids have a significant effect on dyslexia and attention disorders. However, many of these studies have used very low doses of DHA, and often included much more of the twenty-carbon omega-6 ARA, which competes with and inhibits the twenty-carbon omega-3 EPA.

Since hyperactivity is part of some of these behavior disorders, I would like to share another recent article. A Japanese study[11] examined the hyperactivity and anxiety of students during examination time in that country. Those students who were maintained on a soybean oil diet showed increased levels of aggressive behavior, while those taking 1.5 grams of DHA daily showed no such behavior changes during this typically anxiety-producing period. The difference was astounding.

Schizophrenia

A condition characterized by the inability to think clearly, the failure to manage emotions, and an altered state of reality, schizophrenia is often accompanied by delusions. Researcher D. Horrobine[12] has shown that schizophrenia is related to an abnormality in the body's metabolism of fatty acids. Although unable to study the actual brain tissue, he found that there was a decrease in polyunsaturated fatty acids in red blood cell membranes in patients with schizophrenia as compared with people who did not have schizophrenia.

Hormonal, genetic, and environmental components all contribute to schizophrenia. Schizophrenic patients tend to have low levels of DHA in their systems. Preliminary studies have shown that ingestion of 10 grams of a combination of DHA and EPA daily for several months markedly lessened symptoms in schizophrenics for many months.[13]

Other natural therapies for schizophrenia that have been found to be at least somewhat effective include vitamin E, an important fat soluble antioxidant that protects cell membranes; alpha lipoic acid; N-acetyl cysteine, acetile; L-carnitine; coenzyme Q_{10}; phosphatidylserine; NADH (nicotinamide adenine dinucleotide); and ginkgo biloba.

Glutathione is an antioxidant enzyme produced in our bodies that helps support cell membranes and protect cells from oxidative stress. It also seems to lessen some neurologic symptoms of schizophrenia. It's important to note that taking the acetaminophen (Tylenol) greatly lowers glutathione levels because glutathione is needed to bind acetaminophen in order to excrete it from the body. Since low levels of glutathione have been associated with neurologic disease, cataracts, and skin deterioration, taking acetaminophen frequently for pain can actually cause other, more serious problems. The sulfur-containing cysteine can boost glutathione production and is available in supplement form as N-acetyl cysteine.[5]

Alzheimer's Disease

Noted neurologist and author Dr. David Perlmutter has estimated that there may be as many as 4.5 million people with Alzheimer's disease living in the U.S.—and that number appears to be growing.[14] There are indications that low levels of DHA contribute to the increased risk of senile dementia, a category of conditions that includes Alzheimer's disease, organic mental syndrome, and chronic brain syndrome. In the face of this evidence, it may be important for your loved ones or friends who are exhibiting early memory loss or forgetfulness to begin therapy with DHA. There is no way to know if their forgetfulness will progress to a full-scale disorder, but DHA is crucial for normal neurologic function.

Studies have shown that doses of 700 mg and 1,400 mg of DHA taken daily can improve symptoms of both cerebrovascular dementia, caused by insufficient blood flow to the brain, and true Alzheimer's disease.[15] Since we cannot biopsy the brain, red blood cell phosphotidyl/DHA samples are used as an indication of body DHA levels. People with phosphotidyl choline/DHA levels less than 3.5 percent of their total fatty acid levels had two-thirds greater risk of developing senile dementia. Schaeffer[16] reported similar findings—that a reduction in phosphatidyl choline/DHA compound in the blood is associated with an increased risk of dementia.

On the other hand, Masaki and the Honolulu Heart Program[17] found that Japanese-American men in Hawaii who took vitamins C and E were 88 percent less likely to develop vascular dementia.

Other studies have shown that Alzheimer's patients have less DHA in their blood cells; instead, there are high blood levels of DHA breakdown products, including EPA and inflammatory components. In other words, in Alzheimer's patients, the "good" fat is being destroyed—leaving behind inflammatory breakdown products—and it is not resupplied in the body. Thus, the DHA level decreases.

A recent study followed seven of thirty nuns living in the same convent who took multivitamins over their lifetimes. After their deaths, autopsies revealed that the brains of those nuns who took vitamins showed less atrophy than the brains of those who did not take vitamins. Of those who were part of the study, fifteen were diagnosed with Alzheimer's disease; autopsies revealed that these fifteen nuns had very low levels of folic acid. Additionally, the participants with advanced Alzheimer's disease had an approximately 30 percent lower DHA content in various areas of the brain compared with the nuns of the same age without the disease.[18]

As is the case with many other neurologic and cognitive disorders, total body health and appropriate nutrition may help forestall the devastating effects of Alzheimer's disease. Table 6.1 on page 82 lists nutrients that can improve brain function, including memory, and keep the brain active and healthy.

TABLE 6.1. SUPPLEMENTS THAT CAN IMPROVE BRAIN FUNCTION AND MEMORY

Supplement	Recommended Daily Amount
DHA	400–800 mg
Vitamin E	400 IU
Magnesium	500–1,000 mg
L-acetyl carnitine	500–1,000 mg (divided doses)
Coenzyme Q_{10}	120 mg, (divided doses)
B-complex	50 mg, including 400 mcg of folic acid

NOTE: Aside from the magnesium and B-complex, all of these are fat soluble, and will need to be taken with a meal that contains some fat.

Parkinson's Disease

Parkinson's disease is a progressive neurological disease that affects nerve cells in an area of the brain called the substantia nigra. These cells normally produce dopamine, a neurotransmitter that helps coordinate muscle movement. Symptoms of Parkinson's include muscle stiffness, tremors, and a gradual slowing down of movement that may ultimately progress to fixed posture, fixed, stare, and loss of facial expression.

Studies have revealed that the brains of people with Parkinson's have reduced levels of glutathione, an antioxidant enzyme produced in our bodies that helps support cell membranes and protect cells from oxidative stress. In individuals with Parkinson's, glutathione synthesis, which normally occurs in the liver, is deficient—a finding that has led experts to believe that there is an association between liver disturbance and Parkinson's disease. Indeed, researchers[14,19] have demonstrated that intravenous glutathione can improve the symptoms of Parkinson's disease; the intravenous therapy resupplies the brain's needs for glutathione. Additionally, glutathione recycles vitamins C and E, and enhances liver and brain detoxification. In one study, the administration of glutathione demonstrated a 42 percent reduction in disability in Parkinson's patients.

Alpha lipoic acid, a powerful antioxidant that regenerates glutathione and vitamins C and E, is an alternative to intravenous glutathione. Alpha lipoic acid (ALA) is ingested orally, is both water and fat soluble, and is able to cross the blood-brain barrier. ALA is a metal chelator, which means it binds toxic heavy metals—such as mercury, lead, and cadmium—in the body, so the body can eliminate them. Although this has not yet been proved, heavy metals are suspected of contributing to the development of Parkinson's disease. The introduction of supplements coenzyme Q_{10}, NADH, and phosphatidylserine (important to stability of cell membranes and cells' mitochondria) may also be helpful.

Other nutrients may also be helpful in preventing or forestalling the development of Parkinson's disease. For instance, acetyl L-carnitine is important in transporting fat across mitochondrial membranes, and in laboratory animals has demonstrated protection from the disorder. Additionally, vitamins C, D, and E, as well as ginkgo biloba, have been reported to provide some benefits. Finally, essential fats, like DHA, that strengthen cell membranes and improve signal transmission must also play a role.

Sleep Disorders

Recent research has discovered a retinal cell that connects the midbrain and the pineal gland, a small organ buried deep within the brain. The pineal gland secretes melatonin, a hormone that is responsible for regulating our biological rhythms. The release of melatonin, which occurs when our eyes register darkness, is what makes us feel sleepy at night. Because it is important in the conduction of electrical impulses in both the retinal fibers and brain, some researchers believe that DHA can be helpful in treating sleep disorders, as well as other problems related to abnormal melatonin levels, including seasonal affective disorder (SAD) and jet lag.

Other Disorders

The following neurologic diseases and conditions have shown

some improvement with DHA supplementation: bipolar disorders; vascular dementia; organic brain syndrome; stroke recovery; alcoholism; amyotrophic lateral sclerosis (ALS)[5]; cerebral palsy; postpolio syndrome; tardive dyskinesia; and drug side effects.

DHA has also been shown to be helpful in treating numerous abnormalities, including Zellweger syndrome; juvenile neuronal ceroid lipfuscinoses; Refsum's disease; mitochondrial dystrophy; phenylketonuria, or Folling's disease; and adrenoleukodystrophy (ALD). ALD is a disorder associated with loss of vision, swallowing, and speaking, as well as with changes in behavior and insufficient adrenal gland hormones. This was the disease suffered by Lorenzo Odone. His parents treated him with a combination of olive and rapeseed oils, and his treatment inspired the movie *Lorenzo's Oil.* Further research indicates, however, that DHA is more effective than these oils in cases of ALD.

KEY POINTS

- Research has shown that DHA is important to the maintenance of cognitive function, and can also play a supportive role in the treatment of many diseases.
- Low levels of DHA are associated with an increased risk of many neurologic diseases.
- Within two generations, non fish-eating communities may realize very high levels of learning disabilities and other neuropsychiatric conditions because of their low DHA levels.
- Many neurologic disorders arise, in part, due to the loss of conductivity of the neurons in the brain. DHA plays a vital role in nerve structure and nerve conduction in all parts of the brain.
- DHA also plays a role in synapses between nerves facilitating neurotransmitters like acetylcholine (the usual neurotransmitter between brain and neurons), serotonin, and dopamine.

CHAPTER SEVEN

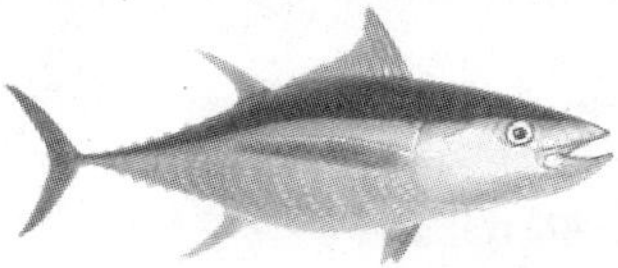

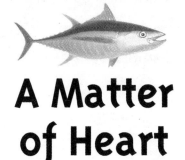

A Matter of Heart

Eating fish is heart healthy, but it's a matter of algae, upon which they dine, that makes the fish fine.

—Doc Abel

The brain is not the only organ that relies on synaptic communication in order to function. It also takes intense communication between cells for the heart to beat in a synchronous rhythm. The heart pumps 200 gallons of blood per day, but it can break down from either physical or emotional factors. DHA is critical for nerve conductivity by virtue of its flexible chemical structure, its ability to conduct nerve impulses and its smoothness as part of the cell membrane that lines all blood vessels.

Several areas of research have indicated that DHA contributes to heart health in a number of ways, such as by:

- Facilitating intracellular communication to prevent arrhythmia
- Decreasing saturated cholesterol plaque
- Decreasing blood stickiness
- Reducing blood pressure

- Reducing heart rate
- Reducing "bad" low-density lipoprotein (LDL) cholesterol
- Increasing "good" high-density lipoprotein (HDL) cholesterol
- Reducing total cholesterol
- Decreasing triglycerides
- Reducing inflammatory proteins
- Relaxing arterial walls
- Reducing stress in general

All of these functions of DHA are important in the face of increased genetic and dietary disposition to heart disease. One hundred years ago, although infectious disease was rampant, heart disease was relatively unusual. Now that infectious diseases are under control, we are facing heart attack (myocardial infarction), stroke, and hypertension as leading causes of death. Heart disease does not discriminate. Although its prevalence in early life is greater in men, it affects both sexes; in fact, a woman's risk of heart disease and sudden death increases significantly after menopause. Of all groups, the incidence of heart disease is highest in African-American women.

Just as it is a major contributor to the erosion of our mental health, stress also degrades our cardiac health. The constant pressure to be responsible and increasingly productive can overwhelm us with anxiety or depression. The physical and emotional torment of stress inhibits breathing, increases our heart rate, affects eating habits, and depletes levels of antioxidants.

If you have history of elevated blood pressure, increased cholesterol, heart disease, or diabetes in your family, or if you experience chronic physical or emotional stress, you should strongly consider DHA supplementation. For one thing, DHA protects against cholesterol plaque formation that can cause high blood pressure, heart attack, and stroke. To understand how this works, let's consider for a moment the differences between two different types of cholesterol: low-density lipoprotein (LDL) and high-density lipoprotein (HDL). Cholesterol circulates in the bloodstream attached to proteins as particles called lipoproteins. LDL cholesterol is known as the "bad" cholesterol because, when it's loaded down with more cholesterol and triglycerides, it deposits this excess on artery walls among other places in the body. Eventually, the excess cholesterol forms plaques, and calcium deposits and platelets collect around the plaque, narrowing arteries. Sudden stress then creates spasms of the coronary arteries, which can cause chest pain, arrhythmia, and heart attack. HDL cholesterol, on the other hand, is known as "good" cholesterol because it has approximately half the amount of cholesterol and triglycerides. Cholesterol has many necessary functions, but plaques in the arteries is not one of them.

DHA also decreases blood pressure. Horrocks[1] showed that unsaturated fatty acids and even the omega-6 linoleic acid can stimulate inflammation in blood vessel endothelium, the lining of the cells. By contrast, EPA has no significant effect on blood pressure. In a controlled study, 4 grams daily of DHA or EPA were given to overweight, mildly hyperlipidemic men. The researchers found that only the men in the DHA group demonstrated decreased levels of both systolic and diastolic blood pressure.

BLOOD VESSEL WALLS

Our modern diet is high in processed omega-6 vegetable oils, which increase inflammatory proteins, free radicals, and "bad" cholesterol—all of which have been implicated in the development of cardiovascular disease. In one noted study, Toborek and colleagues[2] exposed human blood vessel cells to the three different fats: omega-3, omega-6, and omega-9 fatty acids. They found that the omega-6 fats (linoleic acid) increased the inflammation response; by contrast, omega-3 fats (linolenic acid) did not cause inflammation. The omega-9 fats, which are the monosaturated fats found in olive oil, avocado, and macadamia nuts, actually decreased inflammatory activity. Virgin olive oil is recommended as the best cooking oil because it is not fully saturated.

Whether or not you have a history of heart disease in your family, you should begin to include more vegetables, fish, and algal supplements in your diet to maintain optimal heart health. And even if you've recently been diagnosed with a cardiac condition, such as atrial fibrillation, angina pectoris, coronary artery disease, or hypertension, natural remedies remain viable options for treatment. It's possible that many people could considerably decrease their use of medications and still improve blood flow and heart function just by eating the right foods. In fact, in his pioneering books, Dr. Dean Ornish, touts diet and lifestyle modification as the cornerstones of a noninterventional approach to reversing heart disease.

To a patient who had undergone coronary artery bypass surgery four months earlier, I recommended a vitamin supplement regimen including folic acid (in B-complex), vitamin C, vitamin E, and a multivitamin with taurine. Because the patient still noticed skipped heartbeats, I recommended he take additional magnesium at night, and DHA, 200 mg twice daily with meals. Six weeks later, he reported that his skipped heartbeats had vanished, and he felt better. Some of the credit certainly belonged to the DHA.

HEART DISEASE

The correlation between fish consumption and cardiac status has been observed in several large-scale studies, including the thirty-year Western Electric Study.[3] Another trial, published in the *American Journal of Clinical Nutrition* studied the Inuit people in Nunavut, Canada.[4] Those results also showed that a diet high in fish reduced the incidence of heart disease, despite the fact that many of these Native Americans were incorporating Western foods in their diets. Most Americans are consuming at least 20 times more omega-6 fatty acids, often from common vegetable oils (corn, peanut, safflower, and soy oils) than omega-3 fatty acids.

Another study, published in the *American Journal of Cardiology*[5] found a marked decrease in complications after coronary artery angioplasty in patients who were given omega-3 fatty acids compared with those who were not. Furthermore, the Honolulu Heart Study[6] followed 242 patients for approximately 20 years and found a 50 percent *greater* risk in smokers (for those who smoked for twenty years or more) and a 65 percent *reduced* risk in fish eaters (for those who ate fish two or more times per week). Think of the doubled advantage of giving up smoking and eating more fish!

Since it was first discovered that the Eskimos in Greenland or the coastal Japanese rarely died from coronary heart disease, it seemed logical that the thing they had most in common—a diet rich in seafood—may have something to do with heart health. Hughes Sinclair reported in the 1950s the decreased mortality of Greenland Eskimos on a 60-percent fat (essentially polyunsaturated) diet.[7] But when the Eskimos moved to Eastern Canada, the amount of saturated fat in their diet increases, as did their rate of cardiovascular disease. It's clear that we can reduce our risk of heart disease by incorporating more omega-3 fatty acids in our diets, and reducing our heavy reliance on omega-6 fatty acids and saturated fat.

Sudden Death

A major Italian study[8] followed more than 11,000 patients who had survived a recent heart attack. The first of four groups received 2 grams daily of omega-3 fatty acids (EPA and DHA), the second received 300 mg of vitamin E, the third group received both, and the fourth received no supplements. The two groups that received the EPA-DHA combination improved significantly compared with those who took vitamin E alone and those in last group, who received no supplementation. The group that took the omega-3 combination had 20 percent fewer total deaths, 30 percent fewer cardiovascular deaths, and 45 percent fewer sudden deaths, over the course of three to five years. In other words, a high-risk group of people receiving essential fatty acids demonstrated a *decreased* chance of another heart attack, arrhythmia, or sudden death.

Another study, the Diet and Reinfarction Trial (DART),[9] included 2,033 men recovering from documented heart attack, or myocardial infarction. The results of this trial showed that men who consumed fish or fish oil supplements demonstrated an approximately 30 percent reduced mortality over two years compared with those who did not eat fatty fish at least twice a week. The authors suggested that two or three portions of fish per week may reduce mortality in a high-risk group of men.

CHOLESTEROL AND TRIGLYCERIDES: DHA VS. EPA

A major clinical study of men who had already suffered a heart attack showed a reduction of sudden death with DHA supplementation.[10] Patients taking 5,500 mg of omega-3 fatty acids from fish each month showed a 50 percent decreased risk of a second heart attack. These results were astonishing, since the reduction in cardiac arrest was caused by the intake of only 183 mg of both EPA and DHA together per day; also astonishing is the fact that fish consumption did not appear to affect total cholesterol levels. The possibility of being able to reduce the risk of heart disease without reducing total cholesterol levels bore further investigation.

Our first clues came from the data of the Framingham Heart Study.[11] This large longitudinal study first established that cholesterol, particularly the "bad" LDL cholesterol, was a major risk factor predicting cardiovascular disease (CVD). The study also showed, however, that other risk factors such as high triglycerides or low levels of the "good" HDL cholesterol were, in fact, stronger risk factors for CVD. The importance of these latter risk factors was recently underscored with the publication of a large clinical trial of more than 2,500 patients using the cholesterol-lowering drug gemfibrozil.[12] After five years of treatment, in patients who took the drug, there was a 24 percent reduction of fatal and non-fatal heart attack and stroke compared with those who took a placebo. This powerful effect was seen in the absence of any changes in levels of total cholesterol or LDL cholesterol. Instead, there was a 6 percent improvement in HDL cholesterol levels and a 30 percent reduction of triglycerides.

Multiple studies have shown a correlation between supplementation with omega-3 fatty acids and a reduction of triglycerides. One study, in particular,[13] showed a 21 percent decrease in triglycerides in individuals who took 3.8 grams of EPA daily, and a 26 percent decrease in those who took 3.6 grams of DHA daily. Other studies have confirmed that dietary DHA lowers triglycerides, as do fish oil and purified EPA.

DHA supplementation increases high-density lipoproteins—it takes the reaction of "bad" LDL cholesterol and converts it to "good" HDL cholesterol. When oxidized LDL is converted to "reduced" HDL, the cost comes from DHA being oxidized, or losing one double bond, and becoming EPA. Therefore, it's important to note that between 11 and 15 percent of DHA is lost to EPA when low-density cholesterol is converted to high-density cholesterol. You may be wondering why you shouldn't just take EPA, if DHA is going to be converted to EPA anyway. The answer has an interesting twist: As you probably know, a decreased resting heart rate is another sign of good health. Heart rate is reduced with DHA; it is slightly elevated, however, with EPA. DHA has many more positive attributes than EPA. It lowers heart rate, reduces blood pressure, and raises HDL. You don't need to supplement EPA, because it can be created from DHA.[14] Additionally, attempting to raise HDL cholesterol from LDL cholesterol by supplementing with flaxseed will yield very little effect unless very large doses are taken because of the difficulty of converting uphill.[15] Table 9.1 in Chapter 9 presents a graphic explanation of this.

Normally there is an after-dinner increase in triglycerides. A study by Grimsgaard[16] published in the *American Journal of Clinical Nutrition* found that DHA supplementation cuts that triglyceride rise in half, whereas EPA supplementation only decreased that after-dinner elevation by 19 percent. Once again, DHA does the same job as EPA, but DHA does the job much more efficiently.

There is a marked rise in HDL cholesterol and a decrease in triglycerides in patients who eat four fish meals per week (700 mg of DHA per day) or take 4 grams of fish oil (950 mg of DHA) or 1,680 mg of DHA per day without a significant difference between the effects of different supplements.[17] Therefore, my recommendation of 700 milligrams per day is on target for daily DHA supplementation for healthy adults. Supplementing with fish oil is also a beneficial alternative, as long as it comes from a pure source—that is, fish from deep, unpolluted waters—to minimize risk of contamination. It is important to remember that with fish oil as a source of DHA much larger volumes are required.

EAT FISH—AND ALGAE—FOR A HEALTHY HEART

Adding fish to the diet can significantly reduce triglycerides, and some studies have shown an increase in high-density cholesterol. However, studies of fish oil supplementation (using 1 gram or less) show little or no effect on raising levels of high-density lipoprotein cholesterol. High levels of fish oil, as the 4 grams used in the study above, contain more DHA. Why should it be that eating fish improves good cholesterol, yet taking fish oil does not? This mystery was explained recently by a group of international researchers who looked at the effect of the individual components of fish oil.[16] They compared the effects of purified DHA with the other major omega-3 fat in fish oil, EPA. Although both fats reduced triglycerides, the effects on high-density lipoprotein cholesterol were antagonistic. DHA elevated HDL cholesterol, while EPA suppressed it. In other words, the EPA in the fish oil was blunting the positive effects of the DHA. Similar results were seen for the blood-pressure-lowering effects of DHA and EPA. DHA has a component that lowers high-blood pressure, while EPA does not.[14] In considering these results, you may be wondering why we get better results when we eat fish than when we take fish oil. It's simple: Fish had a much higher content of DHA relative to EPA. Fish oils generally contain 80 percent EPA and only 20 percent DHA. Algal oil, which contains up to 40 percent DHA, is a much better source.

Thus, as medical science has progressed we have come to understand the reason why eating fish is good for the heart: the fish oils are important. Furthermore, it is not all the fish oils, but the omega-3 fats, that are important. Finally, now we understand that it is not all omega-3s, but DHA specifically that is the key player. This is why I advise my patients to eat more fatty (cold-water, non-farm-raised) fish when possible. The best sources of DHA are sardines and salmon; caviar and other kinds of fish eggs are also very high in DHA. You may also want to try kelp snacks from your local health food store, or sample a green algae salad or the roll of your choice the next time you go to your favorite sushi restaurant. The paper-thin black wrapping around sushi rolls is, in fact, the DHA-containing algae. (Appendix A lists more good sources of DHA.)

While we're on the subject of sushi: Americans generally cook fish to kill parasites and to make it more culturally tasteful—most of us have not been raised on raw fish and it is an acquired taste that not all acquire. Although cooked fish contains some DHA, cooking (especially overcooking) will break down the cell membranes that contain the DHA itself. Cook fish a little and you lose the hydrogen bonds; cook it a lot and you lose the carbon single and double bonds—that is, you lose some of the protein and polyunsaturated fatty acids.

Because of the absence of DHA in plant-based diets and the human body's limited ability to convert LNA into DHA, vegetarians have significantly lower levels of DHA in serum platelets and mother's milk.[18,19] Vegetarians can get their necessary DHA from supplements derived from algae. See Appendix B for a complete list of supplemental sources of DHA.

KEY POINTS

- Dietary DHA lowers the risk of cardiovascular disease by decreasing blood viscosity, improving blood pressure, increasing HDL cholesterol, and stabilizing the heart rate.
- DHA effectively promotes heart health by reducing pulse rate and blood pressure; other fatty acids do not.
- DHA is twice as effective as EPA in lowering postprandial (after-dinner) trigylcerides.
- DHA improves cardiac rhythm and reduces the chances of sudden death.
- DHA can be supplied from fish, fish oil, or supplements, but is most effective coming directly from eating fish or algae, or taking algal supplements.
- Eating more fish and eliminating smoking improves health as seen in other societies. Reliance on omega-6 fatty acids and saturated fats increases the risk of many illnesses.

CHAPTER EIGHT

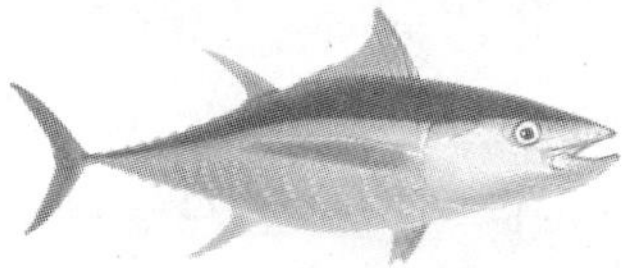

Aging Gracefully

Remembering provides as much pleasure
as being there.

—DOC ABEL

Because researchers have been able to identify some of the critical factors in the aging process, and advances in medical science already have enabled us to live longer, concerns about longevity recently have received a great deal of media attention. In the wake of so much positive news, we can't help but speculate how much better it could get.

Essentially, aging is an accumulation of oxidative stress on all of the systems in our body. Our eyes develop cataracts and experience macular degeneration, our hearing loses acuity, our posture more often than not is less erect, our gait becomes slower and less sure, and our overall energy decreases. No one factor is responsible either for making us age or keeping us young. Still, there are steps we can take to at least keep a toe in the water of the fountain of youth.

Earlier chapters noted that DHA is a major component of brain and nervous system development and maintenance. About fifty years ago, we began to see an epidemic of heart disease; interestingly, this trouble was not accompanied by a similar incidence of nervous system diseases. If our heart problems were brought on by changes in our lifestyle and diet, as I think most experts would agree, why did these changes not also affect the nervous system?

There's actually a very good reason for this: the nervous system was protected in its early development during intrauterine life. The brain and the eyes are almost completely developed and grown to full size in utero. When a baby is born, the head is quite large relative to the body, which is not as fully developed. However, the heart is only one-sixth to one-eighth the size it will be in the adult, and the rest of the body's organs are still growing after birth, too. These organs—the gastrointestinal tract, the skin, the heart, the lungs, and so forth—will tend to show the most abnormalities during the aging process.

The ideal human brain was designed to have a one-to-one balance of omega-3 to omega-6 fatty acids. Disastrously, our diet today features approximately a one-to-twenty ratio in favor of omega-6. In other words, we are overwhelmed by the omega-6 essential fats and are losing omega-3 fats during our lifetime. Since I am speaking of the general population, this of course includes pregnant and/or nursing women. With so little DHA in their own systems, they are not able to pass on this critical fatty acid to their babies, and as a result, brain development and function, along with the entire nervous system, will very likely be impaired. As a population, we are experiencing an increase in the diversity of neurologic conditions, and they are being recognized in children and right on up through the older populations. What we used to call "hardening of the arteries" is no longer the rarity that it once was—all forms of dementia are on the rise. Unless we take action now to restore our depleted supplies of DHA, we will see a continued rise in the incidence of memory loss, distraction, dyslexia, and rage.

Aging is not exclusive to the brain, but involves the body as a whole. For instance, the liver is an important organ for monitoring the body's health. As food comes into the body, chemical substances are absorbed through the gastrointestinal tract and are sent directly to the liver, where they are sorted. Toxins, bacteria, and other particles are removed from circulation, concentrated in the gallbladder, and then excreted as waste. Other compounds are either stored, or are metabolized and sent to the muscles or fat tissue for future use. Some nutritional compounds are combined and are sent to other locations, such as the eyes, ears, heart, and kidneys via the circulatory system. Finally, vitamins are activated by and stored in the liver for distribution, as needed, to other areas of the body.

The big cats on the African plains consume the livers of their prey to get the nutrients that they can't make because they have risen too high on the evolutionary scale.[1] DHA, one of those nutrients, is transported on proteins or bound to phosphatidyl choline to patch cell membranes. But DHA also works on enzymatic reactions in the liver that reduce triglycerides, oxidize cholesterol and affect lipoprotein carriers. Unlike EPA, DHA will raise HDL (good) cholesterol levels.

NUTRITIONAL LINKS TO AGE-RELATED AILMENTS

Evidence is accumulating that certain diseases more frequently encountered in technologically advanced countries can be regarded as nutritionally related. Some of these are: rheumatoid arthritis, multiple sclerosis (MS), cardiovascular and cerebrovascular diseases, hypertension, asthma, and some cancers.[2] The World Health Organization (1982), the Food & Agriculture Organization (1978), and the Surgeon General's Report on Health in the USA (1988) all cite an association between diet and heart disease. Let's take a look at links between nutrition and some of these age-related disorders.

Arthritis

Arthritis is an inflammation of the joints that causes them to become stiff and sore and often swell, as the cartilage between the bones wears down. Through personal experience, I have found that DHA is excellent for arthritis sufferers. Unlike pharmaceutical agents that only relieve pain, DHA builds the strong synovial membranes that line the joints. In the *Journal of Biological Chemistry*, Curtis[3] reported finding that omega-3 fatty acids support chondrocytes that build cartilage and deactivate enzymes that break down cartilage. DHA and other omega-3 fatty acids are also natural cox-2 inhibitors. The "cox-type" enzymes build inflammatory prostaglandins and other compounds that attach cell membranes in joint linings. They work like the nonsteroidal anti-inflammatory drugs (NSAIDS) in your medicine cabinet—without any of the adverse reactions.

It's important to note that, while fish oil and DHA decrease inflammation, the omega-6 ARA does just the opposite. ARA is excellent for building the brain of infants, but high amounts are antagonistic to joints in adults.

Cardiovascular Disease

The inverse relationship between fish consumption and heart disease has been established many times. In 2002, researcher Hu and associates[4] convincingly demonstrated that healthy intake of fish and a high level of omega-3 fatty acids in the diet are associated with a reduced risk of coronary heart disease in women and a strongly reduced risk of death.

Alzheimer's Disease

It is natural to want to keep your memory, but most of us forget things from time to time, and even I . . . now what was I saying? Seriously, the fear of developing Alzheimer's disease is perhaps the greatest fear most of us face about aging. Without our mental faculties intact we feel that we will become a burden to loved ones, and the quality of our daily lives can be reduced to nothing. Are there preventive steps that can allow us to avoid this "worst of all downsides" of growing old? In fact, there are many well-publicized supplements for memory preservation, including vitamin E, coenzyme Q_{10}, magnesium, ginkgo, L-acetyl carnitine, and phosphatidyl choline. Still, not surprisingly, the most basic and best approach is an overall healthy lifestyle and diet.

A 1999 PBS program on aging moderated by Bill Moyers highlighted five factors that enable the elderly to maintain good memory. These are:

1. a changing social environment: socializing with others
2. cardiopulmonary health: avoiding serious heart or lung disease
3. plenty of exercise: walking four to seven times a week
4. fine motor control: for example, using a computer, playing chess, darts, or knitting
5. a flexible personality: the ability to cope with change

You could also add two more factors to this list: the dietary choices your mother made before, during, and after her pregnancy; and your own current dietary habits. With the exception of exercise, all of these factors can be enhanced with DHA supplementation.

As mentioned in Chapter 6, a group of researchers at the Sanders Brown Aging Institute demonstrated that individuals with advanced Alzheimer's disease had about a 30 percent lower DHA content in various areas of the brain compared with the those of the same age without the disease.[5]

A recent Boston University study examined the correlation between DHA status and the development of Alzheimer's disease in approximately 1,200 elderly participants.[6] This population was unique in that it represented a well-studied group of individuals from Framingham, Massachusetts, known as the "Dementia

Cohort." The participants were divided into two groups—a low-DHA status group and a high-DHA status group. Researchers kept in contact with the participants over the course of ten years, routinely checking for any signs of Alzheimer's disease in hopes of identifying risk factors that would predict the onset of the disease. The results showed that individuals in the low-DHA status group had a statistically significant 67 percent greater chance of developing Alzheimer's disease, compared with individuals in the high-DHA status group.

Diabetes

A fourteen-year study of the connection between dietary trans-fatty acid intake and the risk of diabetes in 84,000 middle-aged women found that just a 2 percent increase in trans-fatty acids increased the risk of diabetes by 39 percent. (Remember, these trans-fats are found in margarine, processed vegetable oils, and fried foods, which are making up an increasingly large percentage of our American diet.) The women who consumed more PUFAs than the other women were 37 percent *less* likely to develop diabetes. Such results indicate that by replacing 2 percent of trans-fats calories with PUFAs, you could dramatically decrease your risk of diabetes.[7]

Incidentally, DHA is one fat that will not cause weight gain. You may even lose weight by replacing saturated fats with DHA.

Cancer

Immunity often decreases with age. Diet, environmental factors, infections, stress, and synthetic drugs may accelerate this decline. PUFAs, especially DHA, play a role in rebuilding immunity, since they support organ function and reduce many inflammatory responses throughout the body.

A Colorado State University study showed that fish oil supplementation in thirty-two dogs with cancer significantly improved their survival rate.[8] It is my belief that the EPA/DHA supported healthy cells, helping the body stay strong to fight the cancer, rather than acting specifically on the cancer cells.

Many other studies have also looked at links between cancer and essential fatty acids. For example, Zhu and colleagues[9] analyzed a series of biopsies of breast lumps taken from postmenopausal women. Not surprisingly, they found that women with the highest fatty acid composition of breast adipose tissue had the lowest risk of breast cancer. So we can conclude that essential fatty acid supplementation protects postmenopausal women from breast cancer.

In 1999, Rose and Connally[10] reported in the *International Journal of Oncology* their findings on the role of DHA in suppressing breast cancer cells in mice. They discovered that the DHA molecule inhibits the growth of new abnormal blood vessels, which are necessary to help cancers grow. A 2001 study at Nagoya University School of Medicine[11] showed that, in vitro, a solution of mekabu—a seaweed common in the Japanese diet—was strongly effective in arresting three kinds of human breast cancer cells. In fact, the results with seaweed were more impressive than with a chemotherapeutic agent that is commonly used to treat breast cancer.

In 2001, Swedish investigators published the results of their twenty-one year study on the connection between fish consumption and the development of prostate cancer in 6,272 men.[12] Those who never ate fish had twice the incidence of prostate cancer compared with moderate fish eaters. The authors suggested that this occurred because omega-3 fats from fish compete with omega-6 fats that make pro-inflammatory and cancer-promoting molecules in the body.

DETOXIFICATION AND WEIGHT CONTROL

While we can have the occasional bout of constipation at any age, as we grow older the gastrointestinal tract becomes less efficient and we are more prone to difficulties. Sometimes the body will have trouble absorbing the nutrients from the food that we eat. Other times, things may get, well, stuck.

Believe it or not, studies have shown that various types of seaweed are effective in absorbing toxins like heavy metals from the blood, stimulating the growth of healthy bacteria that we need for digestion, and even improving bowel function. Besides all of this, seaweed is rich in vitamins and mineral salts—especially iodine—that can help control hyperthyroidism.[13] And seaweed has another interesting quality. It contains long-chain sugar molecules called *polysaccharides* that form natural plant gums known as mucilage when they come in contact with water. These distend the stomach without being absorbed, making one feel full, so it can be useful as an appetite suppressant. This can come in handy for those of us who have slowed down a bit and are not as active as we used to be.

DHA assists in numerous other youth-sustaining maintenance tasks in the body, such as muscle and bone development, and lung and colon function; it also improves symptoms of asthma, cystic fibrosis, and attention deficit disorder, and lessens the discomfort of breast cysts. DHA even helps lubricate hair and skin. My 165-pound Newfoundland dog, who consumed only 400 mg of DHA per day, was frequently complimented on the shine of his coat.

The U.S. Department of Agriculture's Human Nutrition Research Center has studied the aging mammalian brain. This center has developed recommendations that have been adopted by academic veterinarians. The role of antioxidants and essential fatty acids have been substantiated by adding them to dogs' diets experimentally. Multiple centers have now already recognized improved mental function in elderly dogs on such fortified diets.

KEY POINTS

- You can age gracefully and hold on to your memory while

reducing the risk and severity of depression by supplementing with DHA.

- Omega-3 fats compete with the omega-6 fats, which make pro-inflammatory and cancer-promoting molecules in the body.

- DHA does not cause weight gain and may work as effectively as your arthritis medication. In fact, you may lose weight by substituting saturated fats with DHA-containing foods.

- It is important to discuss the overwhelming evidence for essential fatty-acid supplementation with your physician so they can incorporate it into your plan of care.

- What we eat, do, and think today may contribute to the maintenance of our cognitive and other body functions for a lifetime.

CHAPTER NINE

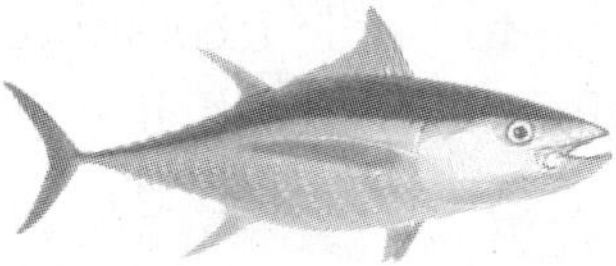

Building a Better Temple: DHA and Wellness for Life

Priority number one is living.
Priority number two is living well.
—DOC ABEL

Genetic factors control much of our development and our innate intelligence. Our tendency to develop certain diseases may be built into our genes, but these diseases will develop only under certain circumstances. Diet is the cornerstone of the broader foundation of health, and nutrition plays a crucial role in maximizing our genetic potential. The gradual depletion of DHA in our modern diet is becoming obvious through the growing incidence of many diseases.

DHA is not a magic bullet, but it is a necessary component of every cell in our bodies. It is critical in all aspects of our health, and nowhere is it more important than in infant nutrition. Our first taste of DHA is provided to us though the placenta. The brain and retina are formed in utero and may still be developing in a premature infant. If a mother does not have an adequate supply of DHA in her body's stores, the child's development can suffer. After birth, babies continue to receive DHA through mother's milk. New mothers who decide to breastfeed should take care to include adequate amounts of DHA in their daily diets; those who choose to bottle feed should select DHA/ARA supplemented infant formulas. As their children grow, parents should make sure that they eat healthy diets and take in plenty of DHA through diet or supplementation; this is especially true for those children with attention deficits, learning disabilities, and tendencies to emotional outbursts.

Let's return, for a moment, to the cell that has been a part of life since the earliest algae evolved. The cell membrane maintains the integrity of the cell, while keeping out unnecessary fluids and materials. DHA contributes greatly to the structure that both supports the cell membrane and, in more advanced organisms, binds cells together. Additionally, no other molecule can claim such efficiency in transmitting nerve signals, smoothing out platelet surfaces, and lining joints.

As we've learned, when our ancestors began to include fish in their diet, their brain size dramatically increased. This major evolutionary development was directly linked to a marine diet and the development of a placenta that selectively concentrated long-chain PUFAs for the growing embryo. Now, unfortunately, the excess of omega-6 fatty acids and the reduction of omega-3 fats in the nutrition of land animals has led to greater body weight without further accompanying brain enlargement.

If we agree that a larger, optimally functioning brain is something worth having—and I think most of us *would* agree—then we'll need to start right now adding more DHA-rich foods in our diets. In this book I've tried to address the various benefits of getting DHA directly from the food we eat rather than relying on supplementation. You now know that some animals can make their own DHA slowly, over a lifetime, by building it from seeds and grains. But as a practical matter, humans cannot produce enough to keep up with either the everyday emotional and mental stresses we encounter, or the wear and tear on our bodies.

The big cats intuitively know that they must eat other animals to build a rich supply of PUFAs. Native Americans lived off the buffalo that ate healthy grains, and fish that fed on algae in clean, unpolluted waters. Our early ancestors ate organ meats because liver and brain are excellent sources of DHA and other long-chain essential fatty acids that are necessary for the brain development. Of course, all animals cannot make DHA from LNA in equal amounts, so the levels found in the livers and muscles of different animals vary widely.

Marine organisms contain an abundant supply of DHA. And algae are the most prolific producers of DHA—after all, life evolved in the seas. Fish are an excellent source of DHA, but fish cannot make DHA for themselves any better than we can. Rather, they get the pre-formed DHA from their diet of the phytoplankton or algae in the oceans. Algae are the mother's milk of the fish world.

The daily average intake of DHA's precursor LNA in industrial populations ranges from 1.0 to 2.2 grams per day. Much of that is contained in products such as unhardened or partially hardened soybean and canola oils. While LNA is also present in chloroplasts of green leafy vegetables, these chloroplasts are difficult to digest, so the bioavailablity of LNA is poor.[1]

Let's examine the various sources from which we can obtain 200 mg of DHA per day. Table 9.1 on page 108 lists five different food sources that, in the quantities listed, each yield 200 mg of DHA.[1]

Although in earlier chapters I touted the benefits of getting DHA from eating fish as a regular part of our diet, I've also pointed out that both our oceans and our soil are being depleted of essential nutrients, and many of the fish that now appear in the markets and restaurants have been farm-raised (and therefore grain-fed) as opposed to algae-fed. As a result, there is a great variability in the amount of DHA available in salmon and other cold-water fish.

Over the past 100 years, having long ago left the tropical

TABLE 9.1. FOOD SOURCES THAT YIELD 200 MG DHA

Food Source and Quantity	DHA Yield
500 mg DHA-enriched algal oil	200 mg
1,000 mg EPA	200 mg
10,000 mg fish oil	200 mg
20,000 mg linolenic acid (LNA)	200 mg
300,000 mg soybean oil	200 mg

shores of our fish-eating existence, it has become increasingly difficult for us to maintain our bodies as the temples they should be. Our dependence on vegetable oil has been growing; while these oils enhance taste and increase shelf life, they provide no antioxidant or cellular support function. Many of us have succumbed to the ease and convenience of prepared and processed foods, consequently adding an increasing amount of saturated fat to our diet. We often eat a quick meal on the run, instead of making up a shopping list or intentionally working our way through the organic grocery aisles at the supermarket. Ironically, here in the richest of all countries, we are experiencing a degradation in health that is not reflected worldwide.

The average consumption of DHA in other countries is remarkably higher than it is in the United States. Typical consumption of DHA in Japan, for example, is about 600 mg per day.[2] A recent USDA food intake survey determined that the average intake of DHA by adults in the US is far less than 100 mg per day.[3] When I formulated my Able Eyes ocular supplement with Carlson Laboratories (see Appendix B), I included 100 mg of DHA along with the other important nutrients for eye health. But surprisingly, despite all that has been revealed about its benefits, DHA is not a component of multivitamins in general.

Of most concern is the low intake of DHA by women of childbearing age—only about 30 mg per day. In 1995, the World Health Organization made it clear that, for women, an adequate

DHA level *prior* to pregnancy is critical to ensure the best outcome when they do become pregnant. And remember, elevating the DHA intake during pregnancy and lactation are of the utmost importance to the lifelong well-being of the child, as well as to the health of the mother herself.

The consensus is that an adequate DHA intake is at least 300 mg per day—ten times the present average consumption level in the United States. Table 9.2 below (which you will probably recognize from Chapter 3) shows the recommended amount of the DHA daily; adherence to a balanced diet is necessary to get the rest of the essential fats. Therefore, during pregnancy, infancy, childhood, adolescence, adulthood, and on into old age, it makes sense to ensure optimal health by supplementing with DHA or DHA-rich foods.

A vegetarian diet, in contrast to an omnivorous diet, is severely lacking in omega-3 fatty acids.[4] Vegan diets do not include fish, fish oils, eggs, or organ meats. Therefore, proper supplementation is extremely important. To cite just one supporting study, in 1996, Conquer and Holub[5] reported in the *Journal of*

TABLE 9.2. DR. ABEL'S RECOMMENDED DAILY DOSAGE OF DHA

Group	Amount Daily
Premature infants	40 mg per kg
Full-term infants	20 mg per kg
0–1 year olds	20 mg per kg
1–5 year olds	100 mg
5–10 year olds	200 mg
10–18 year olds	200–400 mg
Pregnant or lactating women	600–1,000 mg
18–50 year olds	600–700 mg
50 + year olds	600–800 mg
Vegetarians	1,000 mg

NOTE: Always take your DHA with a fat-soluble vitamin and a meal that contains some fat. It is my recommendation to take divided doses when you are taking more than 400 to 500 milligrams per day.

Nutrition that supplementing with algae-derived DHA reduced the risk factors for heart disease in vegetarians.

If you are taking a multivitamin and wonder whether or not it contains DHA, simply examine the label. You'll see that the example in Figure 9.1 below—like most of its competitors—includes many important nutrients, but no DHA.

DHA is an extremely safe supplement, even when taken in high quantities. Volunteers in one study consumed 6 grams of DHA daily without adverse effects.[6] The male subjects of this study did not even experience gastrointestinal disturbances that may occur when ingesting fish oils. Marine DHA oils (Neuromins) have been granted Generally Reliable and Safe (GRAS) approval for pregnant and lactating women and infant formulas.

Fish oil and algal sources of DHA may be equally effective in certain respects, but may not supply the same amount of DHA. Unfortunately, fish and fish oil may be contaminated with toxic metals or may have deficient levels of DHA because the fish were farm-raised on omega-6-rich grains. Only cold-water fatty fishes are high in DHA. These are cod, salmon, mackerel, sardines, anchovies, tuna, herring, and caviar and other fish eggs. See Appendix A for comparative levels of DHA levels in these sources.

DIETARY SUPPLEMENT

Brand Name

MULTIPLE VITAMINS

100 TABLETS
No DHA Contained Herein

Supplement Facts
Serving Size 1 Tablet

	Amount Per Tablet	% Daily Value
Vitamin A	5000 IU	100%
Vitamin C	120 mg	200%
Vitamin D_3	400 IU	100%
Vitamin E	60 IU	200%
Thiamin (B-1)	1.5 mg	100%
Riboflavin (B-2)	1.7 mg	100%
Niacin (as niacinamide)	20 mg	100%
Vitamin B-6	2.0 mg	100%
Folate (folic acid)	400 mcg	100%
Vitamin B-12	6.0 mcg	100%
Biotin	30 mcg	10%
Pantothenic Acid	10 mg	100%
Calcium	20 mg	2%
Iodine	75 mcg	50%
Magnesium	40 mg	10%
Zinc	15 mg	100%
Selenium	25 mcg	30%
Copper	2 mg	100%
Manganese	2 mg	100%
Chromium	25 mcg	20%

Suggested Use: TAKE 1 TABLET DAILY at mealtime.

Manufacturer Name
Any City, USA

FIGURE 9.1. Vitamin Label without DHA.

Since the beginning of the U.S. and Russian space programs algae were understood to be crucial to a self-contained life support system. For space travelers, not only do these one-cell successful colonizers of Earth convert carbon dioxide to oxygen, but they also are an excellent source of food. Algae are an abundant, renewable resource and certain species have been selected for use in supplements for their high percentage of DHA. Neuromins, Carlson's Super DHA, and Liquid Omega-3 are of high quality, as are many of the other algae sources listed in Appendix B.

Over the past 100 years, technology has increased our life expectancy, while at the same time producing conditions that work against a healthy lifestyle. The typical Western diet contains so little DHA that the "temple" that is the human body is not usually as resilient and strong as it could be. A nutritional approach to good health and a high quality of life requires us to reduce our intake of nonessential calories and foods that stress the body. By adding fish to our diets and supplementing with DHA, we can build and maintain a better temple. We want our bodies to be resiliant under stress and to be able to counteract the agents of free radical formation, such as pollution and smoking, and intake of refined sugar and flour, saturated fats and oils, excessive alcohol, caffeine, artificial sweeteners, and artificial colorings.

Table 9.3 on the following page gives some examples of foods that are good for you and foods you should try to avoid. Remember to always do your cooking with monounsaturated oils. Keep in mind, however, that heat, light, and oxygen all accelerate the degradation of these oils, so to ensure the highest integrity and food value, you should buy them packaged in opaque containers and either refrigerate them or store them in a cool, closed cupboard. Finally, if you are not including three weekly servings of cold-water fatty fish, take one of the supplements listed in Appendix B, and if you eat meat, make sure it's free range, not grain-fed.

I hope that I have convinced you of the amazing benefits

TABLE 9.3 HEALTHY AND NOT-SO-HEALTHY FOODS

Healthy Foods	Foods to Avoid
Cold-water fish	Saturated fats, trans-fats
Fruits and vegetables	Excess salt
Organic meats, poultry, and eggs	Products from animals raised with use of antibiotics and hormones
Virgin olive oil for cooking and seasoning	Artificial sweeteners
Nuts and berries	Artificial colors
Whole grains	Refined sugars and flour
Soy and legumes	Processed foods
Wine in moderation	Excess alcohol
Plenty of good, pure water	

of omega-3 DHA. If you follow the suggestions I have made throughout this book, you should experience increased vitality, health, and well-being. With healthy eyes you can look to a bright future, and with a healthy brain, you may actually remember the journey!

Glossary

Adenosine triphosphate (ATP): The molecule built by adding three phosphates to an adenine base. ATP is the major energy storage molecule inside cells.

Adipose tissue: Connective tissue in which fat is stored as globules in distended cells.

Antioxidant: Any substance that can neutralize atoms and small molecules with unpaired electrons; i.e. free radicals.

Arachidonic acid (ARA): The twenty-carbon omega-6 polyunsaturated fatty acid that is necessary for development of the brain and nervous system. ARA is also a source for the production of pro-inflammatory prostaglandins.

Carboxyl: An end group composed of a carbon atom connected to an oxygen atom and a hydroxyl (-OH) group. This is the terminal end of a fatty acid.

Chloroplast: Intracellular organelle that stores chlorophyll found only in plants. DHA is contained in the cell membranes of chloroplasts, which are difficult to digest.

Cholesterol: A fat-soluble steroid made in the liver and adrenal cortex of animals. It is important to several physiological processes and has been implicated in its oxidized form in coronary artery disease. It is more specificallly broken down into such terms as total cholesterol, low-density lipoprotein cholesterol (LDL, the "bad" cholesterol), high-density lipoprotein cholesterol (HDL, the "good" cholesterol), and LDL/HDL ratio.

Choline: A nonessential B vitamin required for fat metabolism and in phosphatidyle choline, a structure component of cell membranes.

Cis-fat: A fat characterized by having all of its side molecules on the same side.

Daily reference value (DRV): The term applied to nutrients such as fat and cholesterol for which no set of standards previously existed. Along with Reference Daily Intake (RDI) values, they are used to determine Daily Value (DV), which is found on the product nutrition label.

Docosahexaenoic acid (DHA): The twenty-two carbon, six double-bond omega-3 fatty acid that supports all cell membranes, brain, heart, and retina function.

Eicosapentaenoic acid (EPA): The twenty-carbon omega-3 polyunsaturated fatty acid with five double bonds. EPA is a major component of fish and fish oil.

Enzyme: A complex protein substance that can act on another molecule to shorten, lengthen, or otherwise alter it.

Essential fatty acid (EFA): Long-chain polyunsaturated fats that are essential for growth and development. They consist of the omega-3 and omega-6 fatty acids and cannot be manufactured from less than eighteen-carbon compounds. Their families are known as structural lipids.

Fat: A multi-carbon molecule that is soluble in fat (organic solvents) but not soluble in water.

Fatty acid: A chain of carbon molecules with a terminal carboxyl group that allows it to be soluble in fat and pass through cell membranes.

Free radical: An unstable byproduct of a chemical reaction that reacts with other molecules in cell membranes and tissues. These unstable molecules react with healthy tissue, dying cells, and even bacteria and cancer cells.

Glycerol: A form of fat consisting of three carbons with three alcohol (OH) groups, capable of being connected to a fatty acid.

Linoleic acid (LA): An eighteen-carbon polyunsaturated fatty acid with two double bonds that is found solely in terrestrial plants. LA is the parent compound for the omega-6 family of essential fatty acids. Also known as alpha-linoleic acid.

Linolenic acid (LNA): The eighteen-carbon omega-3 polyunsaturated fatty acid with three double bonds. LNA is the parent compound for the omega-3 family of essential fatty acids. Also known as alpha-linolenic acid.

Lipid bilayer: Consisting of two layers of essential fatty acids, phospholipids, phosphates, and choline that comprise the cell membranes surrounding every living cell.

Mitochondria: Intracellular independent organelles that produce all the energy for the cell by metabolizing fats, carbohydrates, and proteins. The molecule ATP is produced in mitochondria.

Monounsaturated fatty acid (MUFA): A fatty acid containing one double bond.

Omega-3 fatty acid: A long-chain polyunsaturated fatty acid (eighteen or more carbons) with the first double bond occurring at the number three carbon; a member of the essential fatty acid family originating from linolenic acid.

Omega-6 fatty acid: A long-chain polyunsaturated fatty acid (eighteen or more carbons) with the first double bond occurring at the number six carbon; a member of the essential fatty acid family originating from linoleic acid.

Omega-9 fatty acid: A long-chain fatty acid with a single bond occurring at the number nine carbon. Olive oil is a prime example.

Oxidant: A byproduct of an oxidation reaction that has a free electron requiring neutralization. Another term for oxidant is free radical.

Oxidation: A chemical reaction involving oxygen that can allow the production of byproducts such as free radicals. Respiration (breathing), fermentation, and combustion are all oxidative processes.

Pathway: The direction in which chemical compounds are built from a smaller basic chemical to a more complex derivative.

Phosphatidyl choline: Also known as lecithin, it is composed of two fatty acids, a phosphate group and choline.

Phosphatidyl serine: A structure lipid in the brain composed of two fatty acids, phosphate and the amino acid serine. Its primary therapeutic use is in the treatment of depression.

Phospholipid: A member of the fat family consisting of phosphorus and fatty acids that make up the cell membrane bilayer. Phospholipids play a major role in the structure and fluidity of cell membranes. In the eye, both fatty acids are DHA, and in the brain DHA and ARA are the main fatty acids.

Polyunsaturated fatty acid (PUFA): An unsaturated fatty acid with more than one double bond. Traditionally they are named by the location of the first double bond (which is called omega).

Prostaglandins: Fatty acid derivatives that serve as messengers to cells and blood vessels in the body. There are three families and other related compounds that mediate tissue reactions.

Reference daily intake (RDI): A set of reference values for vitamins, minerals and proteins in voluntary nutrition labeling. These values were previously referred to as RDA (Recommended Daily Allowances).

Synapse: The space between two nerves that allows communication and transmission of signals via biochemicals such as epinephrine, acetylcholine, serotonin, and dopamine.

Trans-fat: A fat characterized by having certain atoms on opposite sides of the carbon chain. This structure is synthetic and not found in nature.

Triglyceride: A glycerol that is connected to three fatty acids.

Unsaturated fatty acid: Any fatty acid with at least one double bond between carbon atoms. Such a fatty acid may have one to six double bonds. In distinction, a saturated fatty acid or trans-fat has no double bond.

APPENDIX A

Dietary Sources of DHA

TABLE A.1. THE AMOUNT OF DHA IN COMMON FOODS

Food	DHA Content
Egg, hard-boiled (1 large)	19 mg
Chicken, fried (2 pieces)	37 mg
Tuna salad (3 oz.)	47 mg
Shrimp, steamed (12 large)	96 mg
Chicken livers, simmered (1 cup)	112 mg
Crab, steamed (3 oz.)	196 mg
Salmon, smoked (3 oz.)	227 mg
Beef liver, fried (3 oz.)	246 mg
White tuna, canned in water (3 oz.)	535 mg
Salmon filet, pink, baked/broiled (3 oz.)	638 mg

From the U.S. Department of Agriculture, Agriculture Research Service. 1999.

TABLE A.2. A COMPARISON OF THE AMOUNTS OF OMEGA-3 FATTY ACIDS IN COMMON FOODS

Food	**Grams of Omega-3 Fatty Acids per 100 Grams of Food**
Fish oil, cod liver	10.968 g
Mackerel, Atlantic, raw	1.401 g
Herring, Atlantic, kippered	1.179 g
Mackerel, Atlantic, cooked, dry heat	0.699 g
Beef brain, simmered	0.670 g
Sardine, Atlantic, canned in oil	0.509 g
Halibut, Greenland, cooked, dry heat	0.504 g
Beef brain, raw	0.500 g
Halibut, Greenland, raw	0.393 g
Tuna, light, canned in water	0.223 g
Shrimp, raw	0.222 g
Tuna, yellowfin, raw	0.181 g
Cod, Atlantic, cooked, dry heat	0.154 g
Cod, Atlantic, raw	0.120 g
Chicken, liver, all classes, raw	0.050 g
Egg, whole, cooked, scrambled	0.030 g

Source: USDA Nutrient Database

Note: This list is far from complete. *All* fish will contain some DHA. Not all—to the best of my knowledge—have been tested for amounts. Try also haddock, menahadin, Atlantic scallops, Pacific oysters, rainbow trout—or any other!

TABLE A.3. COMPARISONS OF THE AMOUNTS OF DHA IN COMMON FOODS

Food	Serving size	Grams of DHA per serving
Fish oil, cod liver	1 Tbsp	1.492 g
Mackerel, Atlantic, raw	3 oz	1.910 g
Herring, Atlantic, kippered	1 oz	0.334 g
Mackerel, Atlantic, cooked, dry heat	3 oz	0.594 g
Beef brain, simmered	3 oz	0.570 g
Sardine, Atlantic, canned in oil	2 sardines	0.122 g
Halibut, Greenland, cooked, dry heat	3 oz	0.428 g
Beef brain, raw	4 oz	0.565 g
Halibut, Greenland, raw	3 oz	0.334 g
Tuna, light, canned in water	3 oz	0.190 g
Shrimp, raw	4 large	0.062 g
Tuna, yellowfin, raw	3 oz	0.154 g
Cod, Atlantic, cooked, dry heat	3 oz	0.131 g
Cod, Atlantic, raw	3 oz	0.102 g
Chicken, liver, all classes, raw (1 unit)	1 lb. ready-to-cook chicken	0.005 g
Egg, whole, cooked, scrambled	1 Tbsp	0.004 g

Source: USDA Nutrient Database

TABLE A.4. LINOLEIC ACID, LINOLENIC ACID, AND DHA CONTENT IN COMMON FOODS

Food	Total Fat (g)	Linoleic Acid (g)	Linolenic Acid (g)	DHA (g)
Caviar	17.90	0.99	0.55	1.35
Herring	12.37	0.18	0.14	1.18
Canned Salmon	6.05	0.06	0.06	0.81
Sardines	11.45	3.54	0.50	0.51
Oyster	4.95	0.10	0.07	0.46
Crab	1.77	0.03	0.02	0.23
Scallops	1.40	0.01	0.00	0.20
Clams	1.95	0.03	0.01	0.15
Mussels	1.95	0.03	0.01	0.15
Shrimp	1.08	0.02	0.01	0.14
Egg yolks	30.87	3.54	0.10	0.11
Tuna, canned in oil	8.21	2.68	0.07	0.10
Tuna, canned in water	0.50	0.00	0.00	0.07
Eggs, whole	10.02	1.15	0.03	0.04
Lobster	0.59	0.00	0.00	0.03
Egg whites	0.00	0.00	0.00	0.00
Mozzarella cheese	17.12	0.36	0.15	0.00
Brie cheese	24.26	0.45	0.27	0.00
Frozen yogurt	3.24	0.06	0.03	0.00
Ice cream	10.77	0.24	0.16	0.00
Sherbet	1.98	0.04	0.03	0.00
Canola oil	100.00	20.30	9.30	0.00
Corn oil	100.00	58.00	0.00	0.00
Sunflower oil	100.00	65.70	0.00	0.00
Cottonseed oil	100.00	51.50	0.20	0.00
Safflower oil	100.00	74.10	0.40	0.00
Sesame oil	100.00	41.30	0.30	0.00
Soybean oil	100.00	34.90	2.60	0.00
Olive oil	100.00	7.90	0.60	0.00
Peanut oil	100.00	32.00	0.00	0.00
Coconut oil	100.00	1.80	0.00	0.00

TABLE A.4. (cont.)

Food	Total Fat (g)	Linoleic Acid (g)	Linolenic Acid (g)	DHA (g)
Palm oil	100.00	9.10	0.20	0.00
Peanut butter	49.98	14.10	0.08	0.00
Almonds	56.53	11.36	0.40	0.00
Cashews	48.21	7.97	0.17	0.00
Peanuts	49.30	15.58	0.00	0.00
Walnuts	61.87	31.76	6.81	0.00
Black olives	10.68	0.85	0.06	0.00
Chocolate candy	10.78	0.86	0.06	0.00
Avocado	15.32	1.84	0.11	0.00
Coconut, fresh	33.49	0.37	0.00	0.00
Soybeans	8.97	4.46	0.60	0.00
Black eyed peas	0.53	0.14	0.08	0.00
Split peas	0.39	0.14	0.03	0.00

APPENDIX B

DHA and EPA Supplement Sources

SOURCES OF DHA SUPPLEMENTS

Carlson Laboratories • 1-800-323-4141
    Able Eyes (eye care formulation; 100 mg DHA)

Jarrow Formulas, Inc. • 1-800-726-0886

Martek Biosciences Corporation • 1-800-662-6339
    Neuromins DHA Chewables
    Neuromins for Kids
    Neuromins DHA
    Neuromins 200
    Neuromins PL
    Gold Minds

New Chapter • 1-800-543-7279

Road to Health • 1-800-388-3818

Solaray (Nutraceutical Corp.) • 1-800-683-9640

Solgar • 1-800-645-2246

Source Naturals • 1-800-815-2333

Natrol • 1-800-326-1520

Nature's Way • 1-800-962-8873

Vitamin Shoppe • 1-212-682-2817

SOURCES OF DHA AND EPA COMBINED

Allergy Research Group • 1-800-545-9960

Carlson Laboratories • 1-800-323-4141

Jarrow Formulas, Inc. • 1-800-726-0886

Natrol • 1-800-326-1520

Nature's Way • 1-800-962-8873

Nordic Naturals • 1-831-662-2852 (Customer Service)

Solgar • 1-800-645-2246

Source Naturals • 1-800-815-2333

Willner's Chemists • 1-800-633-1106

Your Life (Leiner) • 1-800-533-8482

There are numerous other neutraceutical distributors. Ask the salesperson at your local health food store.

Note: *Algae used for DHA production are benign species that have been selected for their high yield of DHA and do not produce toxins.*

APPENDIX C

Recommended Reading

Here are some books that can deepen your understanding of—and appreciation for—the remarkable essential omega-3 fatty acid, DHA. I hope some of these books will inspire you to include more fish and algae in your everyday diet.

DHA: A Good Fat by James Gormley (New York, NY: Kensington, 1999).

Easy Sushi by Emi Kazuko (New York, NY: Ryland Peters & Small, Inc., 2000).

The Eye Care Revolution, by Dr. Robert Abel, Jr. (New York, NY: Kensington, 1999).

Fats That Heal, Fats That Kill by Udo Erasmus (Canada: Alive Books, 1993).

Fresh Water Fish Cookbook by Eileen Clarke (Stillwater, MN: Voyageur Press, 1997).

The Great Sushi and Sashimi Cookbook by Kazu Takahashi and Masakazu Hori (Markham, ON, Canada: Whitecap Books, 2001).

Guide to the Best Supplements for Your Health by Donald Goldberg, Arnold Gitomer, and Robert Abel, Jr. (New York, NY: Kensington, 2002).

Nutrition and Evolution by Crawfod and Marsh (New Canaan, CT: Keats, 1995).

The Omega-3 Connection: The Groundbreaking Anti-depression Diet and Brain Program by Andrew L. Stoll (Boston, MA: Free Press, 2001).

Polyunsaturated Fatty Acids in Human Nutrition, U. Bracco and R. Deckelbaum, eds. (New York: Raven Press, 1992).

Seaweed: A Cook's Guide: Tempting Recipes for Seaweed and Sea Vegetables by Lesley Ellis (San Francisco, CA: Fisher Books, 1999).

Smart Fats by Michael Schmidt (Berkeley, CA: Frog LPD, 1997).

TECHNICAL BOOKS

DHA: A Nutraceutical for New Mothers by D.J. Kyle (Washington, D.C.: American Chemical Society Press, 2002).

Lipids in Nutrition and Health by Michael Gurr (Bridgewater UK: PJ Barnes and Associates, 1999).

Preventive Nutrition by Adrianne Bendich and Richard Deckelbaum (Totowa NJ: Humana Press, 1997).

References

CHAPTER 3

1. Dyerberg J, Jorgensen KA. Marine oils and thrombogenesis (review). *Prog Lipid Res* 1982; 21:255–69.

2. Nelson GJ, Schmidt PC, Bartolini GL, et al. The effect of dietary docosahexaenoic acid on plasma lipids and tissue fatty acid composition in humans. *Lipids* 1997; 32:1137–46.

3. Simopoulos AP, Leaf A, Salem N. Workshop on the essentiality of and recommended dietary intakes for omega-6 and omega-3 fatty acids. *J Am Coll Nutr* 1999; 18:487–9.

4. David J. Kyle, PhD. Personal communication.

CHAPTER 4

1. Kyle DJ (In Press). DHA: A Nutraceutical for New Mothers, American Chemical Society Press.

2. Al MD, Van Houwelingen AC, Hornstra G. Long-chain polyunsaturated fatty acids, pregnancy and pregnancy outcome. *Am J Clin Nutr* 2000; 71:285 S–91 S.

3. Hibbeln JR. Correlation of low levels of docosahexaenoic acid and post partum depression. Unpublished. Presented at ISSFAL, Tscuba, Japan; 2000.

4. Olsen SF, Secher NJ. Low consumption of seafood in early pregnancy as a risk factor for preterm delivery: Prospective cohort study. *BMJ* 2002; 324:447.

5. Hibbeln JR. Fish consumption and major depression (letter). *Lancet* 1998; 351:1213.

6. Makrides M, Neumann MA, Gibson RA. Effect of maternal docosahexaenoic acid (DHA) supplementation on breast milk composition. *Eur J Clin Nutr* 1996; 50:352–57.

7. Anderson JW, Johnstone BM, et al. Breast-feeding and cognitive development: a metaanalysis. *Am J Clin Nutr* 1999; 70: 525–35.

8. Stevens LJ, Zentall SS, et al. Omega-3 fatty acids in boys with behavior, learning, and health problems. *Physiol Behav* 1996; 59:915–20.

9. Makrides M, Neumann MA, et al. Are long-chain polyunsaturated fatty acids essential nutrients in infancy? *Lancet* 1995; 345:1463–8.

10. Birch EE, Hoffman DR, et al. Visual acuity and the essentiality of docosahexaenoic acid and arachidonic acid in the diet of term infants. *Pediatr Res* 1998; 44:201–9.

11. Birch EE, Garfield ES, et al. A randomized controlled trial of early dietary supply of long-chain polyunsaturated fatty acids and mental development in term infants. *Dev Med Child Neurol* 2000; 42:174–81.

12. Mortensen EL, Michaelson KF, Sanders, SA, et al. The association between duration of breastfeeding and adult intelligence. *JAMA* 2002; 287: 2365–71.

13. Simopoulos AP, Leaf A, Salem N. Workshop on the essentiality of and recommended dietary intakes for omega-6 and omega-3 fatty acids. *J Am Coll Nutr* 1999; 18:487–89.

CHAPTER 5

1. Kyle, DJ The Role of Docosahexaenoic acid in the evolution and function of the human brain. ER Skinner (Ed). *Brain Lipids and Disorders in Biological Psychiatry*. London: Elsevier Science BV, 2002; Pages 1–22.

2. Mitchell DC, Gawrisch K, Litman BJ, et al. Why is docosahexaenoic acid essential for nervous system function? *Biochem Soc Trans* 1998; 26:365–70.

3. Abel, R Jr. *The Eye Care Revolution.* New York, NY: Kensington, 1999.

4. Wong TY, Klein R, Sharrett AR, et al. Retinal arterial narrowing and risk of coronary heart disease in men and women. The Arteriosclerosis Risk in Communities Study. *JAMA* 2002; 287:1153–59.

5. Goldberg D, Gitomer A, Abel R Jr. *The Best Supplements for Your Health.* New York, NY: Kensington, 2002.

6. Wang JJ, Mitchell P, Simpson, JM, et al. Visual impairment, age-related cataract, and mortality. *Arch Ophthalmol* 2001; 119:1186–90.

7. Smith S, Mitchell P, and Leeder SR, et al. Dietary fat and fish intake and age-related maculopathy. *Arch Ophthalmol* 2000; 118:401–04.

8. Seddon JM, Ajani UA, et al. Dietary carotenoids, vitamins A, C, and E, and advanced age-related macular degeneration. Eye Disease Case-Control Study Group. *JAMA* 1994; 272: 1413–20.

9. Tillotson A, Hu N, Abel, R. Jr. *The One Earth Herbal Sourcebook.* New York, NY: Kensington, 2001. To contact Dr. Tillotson, Web site: www.oneearthherbs.com; email: alant3@aol.com.

10. Hoffman DR, DeMar JC, et al. Impaired synthesis of docosahexaenoic acid in patients with X-linked retinitis pigmentosa. *J Lipid Res* 2001; 42:1395–401.

11. Dagnelie G, Zorge IS, et al. Lutein improves visual function in some patients with retinal degeneration: a pilot study via the Internet. *Optometry* 2000; 71:147–64.

12. Hoffman DR, Birch DG. Docosahexaenoic acid in red blood cells of patients with X-linked retinitis pigmentosa. *Invest Ophthalmol Vis Sci* 1995; 36:1009–18.

CHAPTER 6

1. Crawford M, Marsh D. *Nutrition and Evolution.* New Canaan, CT: Keats, 1995.

2. Hibbeln J, Salem, N Jr. Dietary polyunsaturated fatty acids and depression: when cholesterol does not satisfy. *Am J Clin Nutr* 1995; 62:1–9.

3. Peet M, Murphy B, et al. Depletion of omega-3 fatty acid levels in red blood cell membranes of depressive patients. *Biol Psych* 1998; 43:315–319.

4. Pawlosky RJ, Salem, N Jr. Ethanol exposure causes a decrease in docosahexaenoic acid and an increase in docosapentaenoic acid in feline brains and retinas. *Am J Clin Nutr* 1995; 61:1284.

5. Perlmutter D. Brainrecovery.com. Published by Perlmutter Health Center, Naples, FL, 2000.

6. Bates D. Dietary lipids and multiple sclerosis. *Uppsala J Med Sci S* 1990; 48:173–187.

7. Tillotson A, et al. *The One Earth Herbal Sourcebook.* New York, NY: Kensington, 2001. Telephone: 302-994-0565; Website: www.oneearthherbs.com; e-mail: Alant3@aol.com.

8. Block, MA. *No More Ritalin: Treating ADHD Without Drugs.* New York, NY: Kensington, 1997.

9. Stevens LJ, Zentall SS, et al. Omega-3 fatty acids in boys with behavior, learning, and health problems. *Physiol Behav* 1996; 59:915–20.

10. Stordy BJ. Benefit of docosahexaenoic acid supplements to dark adaptation in dyslexics [letter; comment]. *Lancet* 1995; 346:385.

11. Hamazaki T, Sawazaki S, et al. The effect of docosahexaenoic acid on aggression in young adults *J Clin Invest* 1996; 97: 1129–33.

12. Horrobine D. Niacin cutaneous flushing as a probe of fatty acid related cell signaling mechanisms in schizophrenia and effective disorders. National Institutes of Health Workshop on Omega-3 Essential Fatty Acids to Psychiatric Disorders. Sept. 3, 1998.

13. Stoll A. Use of DHA in the treatment of neuropsychiatric disorders. Presented at American College for the Advancement of Medicine. Long Beach, CA, Nov. 2001.

14. Perlmutter D. New Advances in Parkinson's Disease. *Townsend Letter for Doctors and Patients.* Pages 52–57, July 2001.

15. Yazawa K. DHA supplementation in dementia. Presented at International Society for the Study of Fatty Acids and Lipids. Barcelona, Spain, 1996.

16. Schaeffer EJ. Decreased plasma phosphotidylcholine docosahexaenoic acid content in dementia. Keeping your brain in shape—New insights into DHA. New York, NY, April, 1997.

17. Masaki KH, Losonczy KG, Izmirlian G, et al. Association of vitamin E and C supplement use with cognitive function and dementia in elderly men. *Neur* 2000; 54:1265–72.

18. Snowden, DA, Tally CL, Smith CD, et al. Serum folate and the severity of atrophy of the neocortex in Alzheimer's disease: findings from the nun study. *Am J Clin Nutr* 2000; 71:993–98.

19. Sechi G, Deledda MG, et al. Reduced glutathione in the treatment of early Parkinson's Disease. *Biol Psych* 1996; 20:1159–70.

CHAPTER 7

1. Horricks LA and Yeo YK. Health benefits of DHA. *Pharm Res* 1999; 40:211–25.

2. Toborek M, Lee YW, Garrido R, et al. Unsaturated fatty acids selectively induce an inflammatory environment in human endothelial cells. *Am J Clin Nutr* 2002; 75:119–25.

3. Daviglus ML, Stamler J, Orecia AJ, et al. Fish consumption and the 30-year risk of fatal myocardial infarction. *NEJM* 1997; 336:1046–53.

4. Dewailly E, Blanchet C, Lemieux S, et al. N-3 fatty acids and cardiovascular disease risk factors among the Inuit of Nunavik. *Am J Clin Nutr* 2001; 74:464–73.

5. Eritsland J, Amesen H, Gronseth K et al. Effect of dietary supplementation with N-3 fatty acids on coronary artery bypass graft patency. *Am J Cardiol* 1996; 77:31–36.

6. Stern MP. Honolulu Heart Study: Review of epidemiologic data and design. *Prog Clin Biol Res* 1984; 147:93–104.

7. Bang HO, Dyerberg J, Sinclair HM. The composition of Eskimo food in Northwestern Greenland. *Am J Clin Nutr* 1980; 33: 657–61.

8. GISSI (Italian) Dietary supplementation with n-3 PUFAs and vitamin E after myocardial infarction: results of the GISSI-Prevenzione trial. *Lancet* 1999; 354:447–55.

9. Burr ML, Fehily AM, Gilbert JF, et al. Effects of the changes of fat, fish and fibre intakes on death and myocardial infarction: the diet and reinfarction trial (DART). *Lancet* 1989; 9:757–61.

10. Siscovick DS, Raghunathan TE, King I, et al. Dietary intake and cell membrane levels of long-chain N-3 polyunsaturated fatty acids and the risk of primary cardiac arrest. [comments] *JAMA* 1995; 274:1363–67.

11. Laio Y, McGee DL, Cooper RS, et al. How generalizable are coronary risk prediction models? Comparison of Framingham and two national cohorts. *Am Heart J* 1999; 137:837–45.

12. Rubins HB, Robins SJ, Collins D, et al. Gemfibrozil for the secondary prevention of coronary heart disease in men with low levels of high-density lipoprotein cholesterol. *NEJM* 1999; 341:410–18.

13. Mori TA, Burke V, Puddey IB, et al. Purified docosapentaenoic and docosahexaenoic acids have differential effects on serum lipids and lipoproteins, low-density cholesterol particle size, glucose, and insulin in mildly hyperlipidemic men. *Am J Clin Nutr* 2000; 71:1085–94.

14. Mori TA, Bow DQ, Burke V, et al. Docosahexaenoic acid but not docosapentaenoic acid lowers ambulatory blood pressure and heart rate in humans. *Hypertension* 1999; 34:253–60.

15. Kyle DJ. The Role of docosahexaenoic acid in the evolution and function of the human brain. ER Skinner (ed), *Brain Lipids and Disorders in Biological Psychiatry.* London: Elsevier Science BV, 2002.

16. Grimsgaard S, Bonaa KH, Hansen JB, et al. Highly purified

docosapentaenoic acid and docosahexaenoic acid in humans have similar triacylglycerol-lowering effects, but divergent effects on serum fatty acids. *Am J Clin Nutr* 1997; *66*:649–59.

17. Agren JJ, Hannienen O, Julkanenk A, et al. Fish diet, fish oil and DHA-rich oil lower fasting and postprandial plasma lipid levels. *Eur J Clin Nutr* 1996; 50:765–71.
18. Reddy S., Sanders TAB, and Obeid O. The influence of maternal vegetarian diet on EFA status of newborn. *Eur J Clin Nutr* 1994; 48:358–68.
19. Conquer JA, Holub BJ. Supplementation with an algae source of DHA increases (n-3) fatty acid status and alters selected risk factors for heart disease in vegetarian subjects. *J Nutr* 1996; 126:3032–39.

CHAPTER 8

1. Crawford M, Marsh D. *Nutrition and Evolution.* New Canaan CT: Keats, 1995.
2. Horrocks LA, Yeo YK. Health Benefits of Docosahexaenoic Acid. *Pharmacol Res* 1999; 40:211–25.
3. Curtis CL, Hughes CE, Flannery CR, et al. N-3 Fatty Acids, Specifically Modulate Catabolic Factors Involved in Articular Cartilage Degradation. *J Biol Chem* 2000; 275:721–24.
4. Hu FB, Bronner L, Willette WC, et al. Fish and omega-3 fatty acid intake and risk of coronary heart disease in women. *JAMA* 2002; 287:1815–21.
5. Prasad MR, Lovel MA, et al. Sanders Brown Study: Regional membrane phospholipid alterations in Alzheimer's disease. *Neurochem Res* 1998; 23:81–8.
6. Kyle DJ, Schaefer E, Patton G. Low serum docosahexaenoic

acid is a significant risk factor for Alzheimer's dementia. *Lipids* 1999; 34:S245–246.

7. Salmeran J, Hu FB, Manson JE, et al. Dietary fat intake and risk of Type II Diabetes in women. *Am J Clin Nutr* 2001; 73: 1019–26.
8. Ogilvie OK, Fettman MJ, Mallinckrodt CH, et al. Effect of Fish Oil, Arginine, and Doxorubicin Chemotherapy on Remission and Survival Time for Dogs with Lymphoma, Cancer. [PERIODICAL?] 2000; 88:1916–28.
9. Zhu ZR, Agren JJ, Mannisto S, et al. Fatty Acid Composition of Breast Adipose Tissue in Breast Cancer Patients and in Patients With Benign Breast Disease. *Nutr. Cancer* 1995; 24: 151–60.
10. Rose DP, Connolly JM. Antiangiogenicity of docosahexaenoic acid and its role in the suppression of breast cancer cell growth in nude mice. *Int J Oncol* 1999; 15:1011–15.
11. Funahashi H, Imai T, Mase T, et al. Seaweed prevents breast cancer? *Jpn J Cancer Res* May, 2001.
12. Terry P, Lichtenstein P, Feychting M, et al. Fatty Fish Consumption and Risk of Prostate Cancer. Lancet, 357: 1764–66, 2001.
13. Guzman, S., Gato, A., Calleha, JM. Departamento de Farmacologia, Facultad de Farmacia, Universidad Central de las Villas, Villa Clara, Santa Clara, Cuba. Anti-inflammatory, Analgesic, and Free Radical Scavaging Activities of the Marine Microalgae Chlorella stigmatophora and Phaeopactylum tripornutum. *Phytother Res* 2001; 15:224–30.

CHAPTER 9

1. DeDecker EAM. Health aspects of fish and n-3 polyunsatu-

rated fatty acids from plant and marine origin. *Nutritional Health.* T Wilson and NJ Temple, eds. Totowa, NJ: Humana Press, 2001.

2. Kyle DJ. The Role of docosahexaenoic acid in the evolution and function of the human brain. ER Skinner, ed. *Brain Lipids and Disorders in Biological Psychiatry.* London: Elsevier Science BV, 2002.

3. Simopoulos AP, Leaf A, Salem N Jr., et al. Workshop on the essentiality of and recommended dietary intakes for omega-6 and omega-3 fatty acids. *J Am Coll Nutr* 1999; 18:487-89.

4. Conquer JA, Holub TJ. Dietary docosahexaenoic acid as a source of eicosapentaenoic acid in vegetarians and omnivores. *Lipids* 1997; 33:341-45.

5. Conquer JA, Holub TJ. Supplementation with an algal source of DHA increases (n-3) fatty acid status and alters selected risk factors for heart disease in vegetarian subjects. *J Nutr* 1996; 126: 3032-39.

6. Nelson, GJ, Schmidt PC, Bartolini GL, Kelley DS, Kyle DJ. The effect of dietary docosahexaenoic acid on plasma lipoproteins and tissue fatty acid composition in humans. *Lipids* 1997; 32: 1137-46.

Index

A

ADHD, 46, 77–79

Adrenoleukodystrophy. *See* ALD.

Age-related macular degeneration, 61

Aggression, 76

Aging, 95–103
  ailments of, 97–101

Alcohol, 56, 75

ALD, 84

Algae, 4, 9–10, 11, 18, 26, 38, 40, 41, 49, 92–94, 107, 110, 111

Alpha lipoic acid, 63, 83

Alzheimer's disease, 5, 80–82, 98–100

AMD, 61–62

American Journal of Cardiology, 89

American Journal of Clinical Nutrition, 88, 92

Anderson, Dr., 46

Antibiotics, 57

Antioxidants, 12, 18, 36, 54–55

Apollo space program, 40

ARA, 24–26, 35, 44, 47, 48, 73, 74, 98

Arachidonic acid. *See* ARA.

Arthritis, 98

Attention deficit hyperactivity disorder. *See* ADHD.

B

Babies, 43–49
  breast-fed versus formula-fed, 46–49, 78, 106
  development, 47–49

development index, 47
diet, 46–49
growth, 47–49
Baby formula, 46–49
Bailey Mental Development Index, 47–48
Best Supplements for Your Health, 55
Block, Mary Ann, 78
Blood pressure, 37, 62
medications, 57
Blood sugar, 56–57
Blood vessel walls, 87–88
Boston University, 99
Bowel function, 101–102
Brain, 27–30, 37, 43–44, 71–84
supplements to improve function, 82
Breast milk, 44, 45–47

C

Calcium, 8
Cancer, 100–101
Candida, 77
Carbohydrates, 8, 9
Carbon chains, 14–17
Carbon, 8
Cardiovascular disease, 88–94, 98
Cardiovascular system, 36–37, 57, 85–94
Carlson Laboratories, 108
Carlson's Super DHA, 111
Cataracts, 56, 59–60
CDC. *See* Centers for Disease Control.
Cell biochemistry, 19–31
Cell membrane, 7–18, 36–37, 106
Centers for Disease Control, 33
Chlamydia, 77
Chloroplasts, 4
Cholesterol, 5, 21, 37, 87, 90–92. *See also* HDL; LDL.
Cod liver oil, 30
Colorado State University, 100
Cones, 51–53, 66
Conquer and Holub, 109
Cornea, 51
Cortisol, 58, 75
Cox-2 inhibitors, 98
Crawford and Marsh, 73
Crystalline lens, 51

D

"Dementia Cohort," 99–100
Death, causes of, 33–34, 41
Demylinating disease, 76
Dendrites, 73
Depression, 45, 74–76
Detoxification, 101–102
DHA, 1–18, 19–31, 33–41, 43–49, 51–69, 71–84
aging and, 95–103

Alzheimer's disease and, 80–82
babies and, 43–49
brain and, 71–84
cancer and, 100
cardiovascular disease and, 88–94
daily dosage, 39, 108–109
depression and, 74–76
development and, 47–49
diabetes and, 63–64, 100
eyes and, 51–69
heart and, 85–94
learning disabilities and, 77–79
molecule structure, 13
multiple sclerosis and, 76–77
neurologic system and, 71–84
organ systems and, 33–41
overall health and, 2–3
Parkinson's disease and, 82–83
postpartum depression and, 45
pregnancy and, 43–49
schizophrenia and, 79–80
sources of, 1–2, 107–108
wellness for life and, 105–112
Diabetes, 63–64, 100
Diet and Reinfarction Trial, 90
Docosahexaenoic acid. *See* DHA.
Docosapentaenoic acid. *See* DPA.
Dopamine, 82
Double bonds, 12–13
DPA, 53
Drusen, 61
Dry eyes, 64–66
Dyslexia, 78–79

E

Eicosopentaenoic acid. *See* EPA.
Enzymes, 5
EPA, 24–26, 34–35, 90–94, 100
Eskimos, 38, 39, 88, 89
Essential fatty acids, 14–15
Eyes, 37, 43, 51–69, 108
definition of, 51–52
diabetes and, 63–64
diseases of, 58–69
lifestyle choices and, 56–57
nutrition and, 54–56
stress and, 57–58
stressors, 54
sunlight and, 56

F

Fats, 8
saturated, 13–18, 22
unsaturated, 13–18
See also Lipids.

Fatty acids, 9, 14–15, 73
classification of, 15–17
intake for adults, 40–41
long-chain, 15–17, 23, 26
short-chain, 15–17
See also Essential fatty acids.
Fish, 3, 19, 25, 26–27, 45, 92–94, 101, 111
Fish oil, 38, 92–94, 100, 110
Flaxseed, 22–23, 26–27, 92
Flour, refined, 5
Food, healthy and unhealthy, 112
Food and Agriculture Organization, 97
Food web, 26, 29–31
Framingham Heart Study, 90
Free-radical scavengers. *See* Antioxidants.
Free radicals, 11–12, 18, 54–55
Freud, Sigmund, 71

G

Gamma linoleic acid. *See* GLA.
Gastric production, 37
Gastrointestinal tract, 101–102, 110
Generally Reliable and Safe, 110
Genetics, 7, 105
GLA, 24, 35
Glaucoma, 62–63
Glutathione, 80, 82
Goldberg, Gitomer, and Abel, 55

H

HDL cholesterol, 87, 90–93, 97
Heart, 85–94
Heart attacks, 89–90
Heart disease, 85–94, 96
Hibbeln, Dr., 45
Honolulu Heart Program, 81, 89
Horrobine, D., 79
Hostility, 76
Hydrogen, 8
Hyperactivity, 79

I

Immune system, 36, 58
Inflammation, 37
Insulin resistance, 37
International Journal of Oncology, 101
IQ, 46–49

J

Journal of Biological Chemistry, 98
Journal of Nutrition, 109
Jung, Carl, 71

L

LA, 23–26, 27–29, 34–35
Lacriserts, 66

Lancet, 78
Lard, 5
LDL cholesterol, 87, 90–92
Learning disabilities, 77–79
Lifestyle choices, 56–57
Lind, James, 30
Linoleic acid. *See* LA.
Linolenic acid. *See* LNA.
Lipids, 9
  structural, 10
Liquid Omega-3, 111
Liver, 97
LNA, 23–26, 27–29, 34–35, 107
Long-chain fatty acids. *See* Essential fatty acids.
Lorenzo's Oil, 84
Lutein, 61, 67

M

Macula, 52
Macular degeneration, 2–3, 56, 60–62. *See also* AMD.
Martek Biosciences Corporation, 40, 49
Martin/Marietta, 40
Meat, 21–22, 27–29
Meibomian glands, 65
Mendel, Gregor, 7
Mitochondria, 12
Monounsaturated fatty acids. *See* MUFAs.
Monounsaturated oils, 111
Moyers, Bill, 99
MS. *See* Multiple sclerosis.
MUFAs, 16–17, 21–22
Mucous, 37
Multiple sclerosis, 67, 76–77
Muscular system, 37
Myelin sheath support system, 77

N

Nagoya University School of Medicine, 101
NASA, 40–41
National Institutes of Health, 34, 45, 53
Nervous system, 36–37, 43–44, 71–84, 96
Neurologic diseases, 74–84, 96
Neuromins, 111
Neurotransmitters, 72, 82
Night blindness, 68
NIH. *See* National Institutes of Health.
Nitrogen, 8
No More Ritalin: Treating ADHD Without Drugs, 78
Nutrition, 7–8, 13–14, 17, 20–22, 25, 46–49, 54–56, 97–101, 106–112
Nutrition and Evolution, 73

O

Odone, Lorenzo, 84

Omega fats, 16–17
one-to-one ratio, 20, 31, 96
pathways, 23–26
Omega-3 fatty acids, 1, 3, 13, 16–18, 20–31, 33–41, 53–54, 63, 67, 68, 73, 74, 79, 87, 88, 91, 93, 96, 103, 106, 109, 112
Omega-6 fatty acids, 3, 16–18, 20–31, 33–41, 53, 73, 74, 77, 79, 87, 88, 96, 98, 103, 106, 109
Omega-9 fatty acids, 16–18, 87, 88
Optic nerve, 62
Optic neuritis, 67–68
Organ systems, 33–41
Oxidants. *See* Free radicals.
Oxidation, 12
Oxidative stress, 11, 95
Oxygen, 8
bad, 10–13
good, 10–13

P

Parkinson's disease, 82–83
Pathways, 23–26, 29, 35
Perlmutter, David, 80
Phospholipid, 53
Phosphorous, 8
Phosphotidyl choline, 53, 66
Photoreceptors, 52–53, 66, 68
Phytoplankton, 3
Pineal gland, 83
Placenta, 44
Plankton, 26
Polysaccharides, 102
Polyunsaturated fatty acids. See PUFAs.
Postpartum depression, 45
Pregnancy, 43–49
Proclear, 66
Proteins, 8, 9
PUFAs, 16–17, 21–22, 25, 31, 100, 106, 107
Purdue University, 46

R

Retina, 51–53, 55–56, 59–60
Retinitis Pigmentosa, 66–67
Rhodopsin, 52–53
Rice, white, 5
Rickets, 30
Rods, 51–53, 55–56, 60, 66, 68
Rose and Connally, 101

S

Saligan, 66
Salt, 5
Sanders Brown Aging Institute, 99
Saturated fats. *See* Fats, saturated.
Schizophrenia, 79–80
Scurvy, 29–30
Seaweed, 93, 102

Short-chain fatty acids. *See* Fatty acids.
Sjögren's syndrome, 65
Skeletal system, 37
Sleep disorders, 83
Straight chain fatty acids. *See* Fatty acids.
Stress, 57–58
Substantia nigra, 82
Sudden death, 89–90
Sugar, refined, 5
Sulfur, 8
Sunlight, 56
Supplements, 82
Surgeon General's Report on Health in the USA, 97

T

Tillotson, Alan, 77
Trans-fatty acids, 17
Triglycerides, 5, 21, 90–92

U

Ultraviolet rays. *See* UV rays.
United States Congress, 5
United States Department of Agriculture's Human Nutrition Research Center, 102
University of Delaware, 21
University of Kentucky, 46
Unsaturated fats. *See* Fats, unsaturated.
UV rays, 56

V

Vegetable oils, 5
Vitamin A, 61
Vitamin B_{12}, 63
Vitamin C, 30
Vitamin D, 30
Vitamin E, 61
Vitamins, 7, 63, 81, 110

W

Water, 55
Weight control, 101–102
Wellness for life, 105–112
Wesson, George, 5
Western Electric Study, 88
"White thieves," 5
WHO. *See* World Health Organization.
World Health Organization, 39, 97, 108

Other Books from Basic Health Publications

DR. EARL MINDELL'S NATURAL REMEDIES FOR 101 AILMENTS

Earl Mindell, R.Ph, Ph.D.

Recipes for Healthy Living

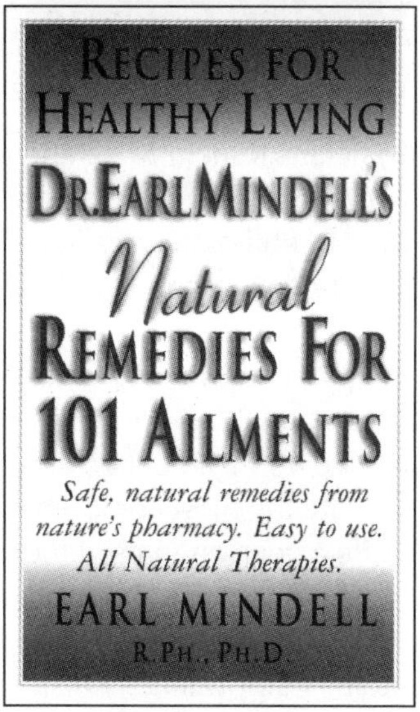

Stop turning to potentially harmful prescription and over-the-counter medicines to ease whatever ails you. Turn instead to Mother Nature for safe, natural, and effective remedies to relieve you of troublesome health conditions. Let world-renowned health expert Dr. Earl Mindell show you how you can use nutritional and herbal supplements to treat common ailments, both large and small. Listen also to his commonsense advice and preventive strategies, and you will soon discover that the symptoms that have been plaguing you are fading. Not only will you feel better physically, but you'll also rest well knowing that you arrived there naturally with nonprescription alternatives.

Dr. Earl Mindell's Natural Remedies for 101 Ailments features the doctor's favorite time-tested recipes for the treatment of various disorders, including allergies, arthritis pain, backaches, colds and flu, dandruff, depression, diabetes, fatigue, fibromyalgia, heartburn, insomnia, jet lag, nausea, PMS, psoriasis and eczema, sprains and strains, memory loss, vertigo, weight loss, yeast infections, and many more!

You'll find yourself turning to this book time after time to learn what you can do to live a healthy and pain-free life like nature intended.

About the Author: Earl Mindell, R.Ph., Ph.D., is an internationally recognized expert on nutrition, drugs, vitamins, and herbal remedies. He is a professor of nutrition at Pacific Western University. In addition to writing several hundred articles on the subject of alternative health, Dr. Mindell has written more than forty books and booklets, including the best-selling *Dr. Earl Mindell's Vitamin Bible* and *Dr. Earl Mindell's Herb Bible*. Dr. Mindell received his pharmacy degree from North Dakota State University and his doctorate in nutrition from Pacific Western University.

Trade Paperback • $19.95 • 224 pages • $5\frac{1}{2}$ x $8\frac{1}{2}$ • ISBN: 1-59120-028-8